HEART AND SOULS

Surviving A Heart attack

Andy Keen

KDPublishing

To: Martha, Gregory & Harry

Prayer is not asking. It is a longing of the soul. It is daily admission of one's weakness. It is better in prayer to have a heart without words than words without a heart.

MAHATMA GANDHI

CONTENTS

PROLOGUE

All the events, details, people and places described in this book are true and real. Everything happened. Some people's names have been changed, some places and people have been deliberately kept vague. But everything is true. Exercise can take many forms and everyone can do something. For your heart's sake, do something.

1 THE LONGEST NIGHT

I was at work and we were busy. It was two weeks before Christmas and tonight was the works Christmas meal and party. Suddenly I started sweating, felt quite breathless, got pins and needles in my left arm and my chest felt tight. But I could still stand, and the pain wasn't that bad; none of my colleagues were nearby to tell anyway. I put it down to working too hard. I resolved to work less hard.

That did the trick. I soon felt better, thought no more of it and went out for the meal that night. I do like my food. The next day at work passed without incident. But when I got home, the same feelings came again and I was just sitting watching TV on the settee. Without knowing what it was that was wrong with me, I just knew something was. But it was a Saturday night, the GP was shut till Monday and you can't just go calling ambulances out, particularly as I knew I'd feel fine again in a few moments. Anyway, it couldn't be a heart attack, I'd seen Eastenders. I'd be clutching my chest, collapsing on the floor and screaming in pain. So that was ruled out. I was also only 43. Nobody has a heart attack at that age.

In the circumstances, I did what any sane, rational person would do. I texted a friend. They told me to call an ambulance. I said I couldn't as I was already feeling better. So they suggested calling NHS direct. If they said to call an ambulance, it wasn't my fault. Finally, I had a plan.

"Hello, you're through to NHS Direct. Are you calling about yourself or someone else?"
"Myself."
"OK. Are you conscious and breathing?"
"Err. Yes."
I explained my symptoms and that I was actually feeling much better already.
"Has this happened before?"
"Well, just once."
"What did you do then?"
"Carried on."
"You didn't seek any medical advice?"
"No." Don't try to make me look stupid. I didn't know it was going to happen again. Anyway, I'd already paid for the meal that night.
"OK. Can you sit down without leaving the phone?"
"Yes. I can manage that."
"OK. Without standing up again, can you reach an aspirin?"
NO! Of course I can't reach an aspirin. Who keeps aspirin in reach of their settee? But "No" is all I actually said.
"OK. There's an ambulance on its way to you. Please remain seated till the paramedics arrive."

Within a few minutes, two paramedics were at the door. They hadn't actually come in an ambulance, but a car. They were laden down with equipment though. I was impressed with the range of things they had. They made me sit down then wired me up to an ECG machine. I was even more impressed they had an ECG machine with them. If you don't know what an ECG is, they place various stickers to your body, then connect wires to the stickers, then connect the other end of the wires to a machine which draws a graph of what your heart is doing. As there are so many stickers, it takes some time to place them all and they always miss at least one when they take them off too. Because there are so many wires, they always get tangled so it takes some time to untangle them. The result is that it takes far longer to set it all up than it does to perform it. To justify this, they did three tests.

They looked at me and said, "You're perfectly normal at the moment."
"That's the nicest thing anyone has ever said to me."
"But," they continued, there's always a but, "the readings do show unusual things. We think you need to go to A&E, if not tonight then first thing tomorrow. In the meantime, don't do anything strenuous." Finally, advice I could follow. "But, as you're not ill now, we can't send you in an ambulance."

I rang my friend, the one whose advice I followed in calling the NHS, and explained.
"I'm on my way," said Kristyan. "I'll bring Becky too. Then I can take you to A&E whilst she looks after your kids." I had a chauffeur, chaperone and babysitter all in one call.

You hear many horror stories about A&E on Saturday nights. Fights, assaults, swearing and the patients can be even worse. But we got there to find peace and tranquillity. Not many people in the waiting room and only one person in front of us checking-in. The person on reception was secured behind glass. It appeared to be sound-proof glass. A few minutes of shouting at each other revealed I was on their system, but under my old address. Once I'd passed my personal details over at a volume everyone in the hospital could hear, we took a seat.

Kristyan got his phone out, opened the camera and took a photo of me.
"Something to remember you by," he said. That cheered me up no end.

To pass the time we played a game of 'guess what everyone

else is here for.' There was a woman standing up despite a lot of empty chairs. I went for haemorrhoids. There was a woman shouting. Kristyan went for laryngitis. The trouble with this game of course, is that you don't know if you're right or not.

Mind you, it can only be a matter of time before privacy laws reach the stage that calling out your name in hospital breaches them. Then the game will be much more fun if the nurse has to say,
"The person with an ingrowing toenail." It will solve who wins.

We were called in to a side room. A quietly spoken doctor was waiting there. He said a few things so quietly I couldn't hear him, then left the room. I looked at Kristyan.
"What did he say?" I asked, "I couldn't hear him."
"Me neither," replied Kristyan.
"So glad you're here."
A nurse then came in through a door, which we hadn't noticed, at the rear of the room behind a curtain.
"Is the Doctor here?"
"Ain't nobody here but us patients," replied Kristyan. He was enjoying himself too much.
The Doctor did come back and gestured we should wait back in the waiting room, so we did.
Not too long after, a nurse came through from the main A&E area,
"Andrew Keen."
"That's us!" shouted Kristyan.
"What? Both of you?" asked the confused nurse.
"No, just him. I'm his carer," said Kristyan, genuinely thinking he was being both helpful as well as funny.
"Well come through," said a confused nurse.
As we got through the doors, a patient, who had just been discharged, was sick all across the floor.

"You'd better go and wait in reception again," said the nurse to us. So near, yet so far.

Not too long after, we were called back through. We followed the nurse and took care to avoid the freshly mopped area of floor. As they were suspecting a heart attack, they didn't make us wait in the next area, so we leapfrogged straight through to a bed. There, they lost no time in taking copious amounts of blood and giving me an almost, but not quite, dissolved aspirin. They did more ECGs too, finding a sticker the paramedics had left on. Soon a cardiac nurse came back to deliver the results of the blood tests. I had indeed had two heart attacks. I was to stay in bed and not move. If I needed the toilet, I was to tell them and they'd get the commode.

I hadn't wanted the toilet, but somehow the mention of the word commode suddenly made me want to go. I could imagine nothing worse than having to use a commode at all, apart from having to use one in an A&E cubicle. And having to use one in an A&E cubicle with Kristyan watching. I put mind over matter and tried to pay attention to the nurse. They were going to admit me and do further tests. It was time to brave the hospital gown.

The hospital gown has to be the worst garment known to man. Although all vital human organs are located at the front of the body, the gown only opens at the back. And open it does. It provides no decency at all. In short, the hospital gown was invented by a pervert with a bottom fetish.

More tests were done on my blood, which only seemed to confirm what they already knew. So they gave me some more pills. They also wired me up to a heart monitor. This was to be my constant friend for the next three weeks. In a surprise move, they also sent me for an x-ray. A porter came and for a brief moment I was allowed the freedom to get off the bed and into a wheelchair. I was taken to the x-ray room where I was asked if I could stand.

"I've stood lots of times and never had a problem," I said, not really understanding the need for the question. It seemed to cheer up the x-ray person a lot though. But then being in a windowless room on a Saturday night can't be all that much fun. You have to take whatever entertainment you can get, I guess. The x-ray showed a sticker left from my last ECG. I was wheeled back to my A&E bed and not allowed the joy of standing again. Too much stress on the heart.

Various doctors, nurses, and other medical people came to look at me. I couldn't eat or drink, but the trolley with food and drink came past regularly anyway and kept Kristyan supplied instead. In the end, it was a porter who came to take me to the ward. I knew this because he said

"I'm going to take you to the ward. I'm only a porter. I need to get a nurse to come too. Just in case." In case of what wasn't explained. I didn't like to ask. I could only hope Kristyan didn't take it upon himself to ask either.

So we set off; me in a bed, a porter pushing the bed, Kristyan walking by my side and a nurse just in case. We arrived at the ward. They let us in but made Kristyan wait outside. It was probably outside visiting hours; it was 1 o'clock on Sunday morning by now. I suddenly felt very alone and a little bit scared.

2 ALL HEART

The ward was unusual in that the nurses' station was in the centre of the room. Round the edge of the room were the beds. This did mean there was always some activity to watch. Although I knew this was a cardiac ward, what I didn't know at the time was that this was a ward where they put you when they weren't sure what to do with you just yet. A holding ward if you like, although assessment ward is the term they used.

It didn't occur to me till afterwards, that there was no TV or anything to do. Your entertainment was restricted to what was happening at the nurses' station and in the surrounding beds. What was happening in the surrounding beds when I arrived, was the occupants being awoken in the middle of the night by a new arrival. I felt a bit sorry for them. It didn't help that a nurse was talking to me and going through my notes.
"So, you've had a heart attack?"
"Yes."
"Have they given you an aspirin?"
"Yes."
"Okay, I'll just do a quick ECG."
She actually removed all the stickers.
"You're not allowed out of bed. If you need anything push this button here." She showed me a remote control that was tantalisingly out of my reach from the bed. It was a big orange button with a picture of an old-fashioned nurse on it. "If you

need the toilet we will bring the commode over. Remember to draw the curtains."

I was fairly sure I'd remember.

"What do you want for lunch tomorrow? The menu is here." I'm not used to choosing any meal in the middle of the night, least of all one still 12 hours away. But there was a roast dinner option so I went for that.

"The light switches are on the same remote control as the call button."

"The one I can't reach."

"Try to get some sleep. The doctors will be around in the morning." With that, she passed me the remote and disappeared. I was wondering which switch to press, without lighting up the whole ward, when I heard a familiar voice.

"Hi mate." It was Kristyan. "They left me standing at the door! Anyway, they said I could come in to say goodbye. So goodbye."

"Yeah. Cheers. Thanks for coming over and bringing me here." I meant it, "and thank Becky for babysitting."

"I will."

"One last thing…"

"Yeah?"

"Can you call my mother and tell her. Not now, no point now. But in the morning?"

"Of course."

"Cheers. Bye."

"Bye."

And with that, he went. He hadn't asked for mum's number, but he can be quite resourceful when he puts his mind to it. I turned several more lights on before managing to get all mine off. Then settled down for minutes of uninterrupted sleep.

When I woke the next morning, or technically the same morning, I thought I'd lost my grasp of the English language. The man in the bed next to me was talking to someone, but I couldn't understand a word. It turned out he was a Polish lorry driver who had suffered a heart attack over here. Fortunately, like me, not a too serious one, and it hadn't resulted in an accident. He was on the phone, presumably home. His English wasn't that good, but considerably better than my Polish. They had to get an interpreter in when the nurses and doctors talked to him. The rest of the time a mixture of mime and charades got us all through. Come to think of it, he might not have been a lorry driver at all. Maybe the mime I thought was him driving a lorry was him milking a cow. Although it's a long way to come to milk a cow.

The last act of the night shift each day is to serve breakfast. This does make an early start to the day, particularly for those of us that had a very late night. But with drinks, cereal and toast, it's worth waking up for. Not too long after breakfast, the ward door opened and in strolled my mother. As she doesn't drive, my aunt and uncle were with her too. I related the story of how I'd ended up there. Then, the refreshment trolley came round. I do like my food. There was a selection of snacks and drinks to choose from. I had a banana and a coffee. After that the doctors came round and Mum left. Both Mum and the doctors said they'd see me again tomorrow.

They were going to keep me in longer, I wasn't allowed out of bed and I'd be moved into a proper ward. This was the general agreement in the assessment ward. But in the meantime, they gave me some more pills. As it was a cardiac ward, no one could get out of bed, so we all enjoyed a silver service lunch, served in bed. You know it's mealtime as a big trolley is wheeled onto the ward, smelling of food. No particular food, just food.

This hot trolley contains all the meal options for that mealtime. There's enough of each dish for everyone who ordered it. The nurses plate it up and put the plate on a tray with cutlery and condiments. It seems odd that we can't get out of bed, but are given salt. They also put a container of fruit juice on the tray; this is served in a plastic round container, which is impossible to drink out of without spilling it down you.

Pudding is also served on the tray at the same time. A complete meal, on one tray. A lot of jokes are made about hospital food, but I found it very nice. And they certainly don't let you go hungry. As well as your three meals, the snack and drink trolley comes round between breakfast and lunch and again between lunch and dinner. Then there is the bedtime drinks trolley for anyone who is still peckish.

Sunday afternoon passed with more visitors. My children brought me in a radio to try and prevent boredom. A friend, who is a doctor, dropped by too. Although cardiology isn't their area of expertise, they were able to answer some of my medical questions and explain words I'd heard mentioned. Why call a spade a spade when you can call it a garden digging implementation tool for the purpose of creating holes? Doctors like to use more words than are strictly necessary.

After dinner, a porter came to move me onto a new ward. I don't really know the difference being on a different ward makes, but it seems to matter to them. I was wheeled off to my new home, accompanied by a nurse, just in case.

On the new ward, the layout was pretty much the same as on every hospital ward. There was a nurses' station, a few bays of 6 beds and a few single rooms. Being a heart ward though, the nurses' station had a bank of monitors, one for each patient, relaying their heart beats and pulses, all seen in one glance. Every so often, one would flash and beep loudly if the heart rate wasn't within the set parameters. As this happened so often, no one batted an eyelid.

I was given a single room. It was en-suite. But I couldn't use it as I wasn't allowed out of bed. Instead they left cardboard bottles to go in. I could also ask for the commode if needed: how thoughtful. There was a TV in the room and a remote control attached to the bed. From this, I could summon a nurse, turn the light above my bed onto three different settings or even off. It also tilted the bed into various positions, controlling feet and head ends independently. Some positions even a contortionist would struggle to get into. But it didn't control the TV.

Kristyan came to visit me. He had hours of fun playing with the bed controls, very nearly tipping me out Wallace & Gromit style when he pressed the vertical button. Why a patient needs to be tipped out of a bed feet first I never did understand, or want to find out. What I quickly learned was to ensure that when the last visitor of the night left, they had to leave me set up for the night. TV on the right channel for that nights viewing, windows open enough for air, but not too wide for a draught, remote within my reach, blinds drawn and the light switches by the door in the correct positions.

The light switches were the most problematic. I could control the light above my bed perfectly well from my remote; this created enough light for my needs, but during the day various staff would turn the room lights on, so they needed turning off each evening. There were two switches, one unmarked and one marked 'day' at the top and 'night' at the bottom. Between them they created various options.

With the blank switch down and the other on 'day', this gave full lighting. With the blank switch up and the other on 'night', this left a couple of lights on dim by the door. But with the blank switch up and the other on 'night', this dimmed all the lights and with the blank switch down and the other on 'night', this made the two lights by the door turn on full. It took several attempts over several days to work this out. If someone had been in the en-suite and left the light on, that illuminated round the door, which would be unnoticed till the lights went out. But to then switch the en-suite off, you'd have to turn the lights back on, then start the whole maddening switch off procedure again.

The first act of the night shift when they come on duty is to dispense medication. I was up to six tablets at night now, including the almost dissolvable aspirin. This means, of course, you can't go to sleep too early. After medication, you can settle down. But not for long. The night shift check on you during the night by taking your blood pressure and temperature, then apologising if they woke you. Then they wake you before they go home to give you breakfast.

3 BACKWARDS & FOUR WARDS

And so I settled into the daily routine. Wake for breakfast in bed (I had coffee, Rice Krispies, two rounds of toast with butter and marmalade, since you ask.) Then they come round with a bowl of water, cloths, soap, razor, toothbrush, toothpaste and towel. I was allowed out of bed to wash. Only to the chair next to the bed, but still, out of bed is out of bed. During this time, they too made the most of it by changing the bed.

The toothpaste tube contained enough exactly, and no more, to clean your teeth once; and once only. If you've ever wondered what toothpaste tastes like if it's not flavoured minty, then the NHS have the answer for you. It's disgusting.

Whilst bringing the new bedding, they'd bring new pyjamas too. Although slightly better than a hospital gown, hospital pyjamas use press-studs as the only fastenings, so you can regularly come unpopped at inopportune moments.

Then the refreshment trolley. Lunch. Refreshment trolley. Visitors. Dinner. Visitors. Drinks. Medication. Bed. Repeat. It's easy to get in the routine. All the while wired up to a heart monitor. Although never moving, the wires still managed to get tangled. Every time you'd have to attempt to untangle yourself. Every time you'd have to call for assistance.

They had small pots of custard on the refreshment trolley. I started having those with my banana. I'd wanted to chop the banana up and put it the pot, but there were no knives, only spoons. In the end I used the banana as a scoop to eat the custard. Not dignified, but the best I could do.

Occasionally, in a break to the routine, they'd take you off for a test or procedure. This could either be a welcome break to the routine, or an unwelcome intrusion into the routine, depending on what they were doing. One day I went for an
x-ray; that was a nice trip out. Other days were less good.

Quite often these trips were unannounced. The first I'd know about them was when a porter turned up to take me out. I'd therefore often have no idea what was going to happen when I got there. So it was when I went for an angiogram.

I was taken down in my bed and placed in a waiting area of beds. Those who were coming for the procedure as an out-patient still had to get into a bed. As I still had no idea what was going on, I asked a nurse.
"You're going to have an angiogram," she said, as if that explained it.
"Speak to me like I'm five and tell me what is going to happen."
"Well, we get a very long needle and insert it into your wrist, or some doctors prefer the groin, and then thread it through your veins and round your heart. Meanwhile an x-ray machine above you shows the doctor what is happening and if your arteries are blocked. If they are, they may be able to pop a stent in-basically something which opens the arteries back up-if really blocked you have to have bypass surgery."
"Thank you. Doesn't it hurt having a needle going round your veins?"
"No. There are no nerves in your veins, so you can't feel it."
"Are you sure?"
"Oh yes. You can always ask for painkillers if it's uncomfortable anyway."
"Why would I need painkillers if it doesn't hurt?"

Before she could answer that another nurse turned up.
"Excuse me, we have a student nurse here today. Would you mind if they did the initial injection as they haven't done one before?"
"Err, I guess so."

As it happened, a 'more interesting' case turned up so the student went to them instead. I can't pretend I was disappointed. I was given an injection and a canular, inserted by a fully qualified nurse, and wheeled through to the treatment room.

I was nervous, so I was shaking involuntarily a bit. The doctor said,
"We will give you something to relax you."
As soon as it was administered, my body couldn't move. It was like the scene in Johnny English where he accidentally injects the muscle relaxant. Still, it did the job. I lay motionless. I looked around. To my left was a bank of screens all ready to show my insides. Above was a small x-ray machine. The nurse asked me to hold out my right arm at right angles to my body. They slid an extension to the bed under it to keep it up. Then in went the needle. I shut my eyes.

To be fair, that bit didn't hurt. But where it went in and the unusual angle my arm was being twisted and turned into, meant that my arm did hurt. A lot. I didn't want to make a fuss or sound like a wimp though.
"Everything OK?"
"Oh yes. Fine," I lied.
"Err, actually my arm does hurt a bit." Better to be honest. "Just a bit." No need to appear a wimp.
"No problem. We will give you some painkiller."
Instantly, I could feel it coursing through my veins. It felt cold, particularly for a part of the body that had no nerves. The pain went. Almost straight away replaced by the feeling of nausea.

"Excuse me, sorry to be a pain, but I do feel a bit si...." Before I'd finished the word, let alone the sentence, a cardboard sick bowl was in front of me. If you ever want to see medical staff move at lightening speed just say that you feel sick. It's part of their training to have a sick bowl in front of you in under half a second.

I wasn't sick and I didn't have stents either. There were three blockages they could have stented, but two they couldn't. As they were going to have to open me up to do a bypass on them, might as well do all five. A quintuple bypass it was.

Just to be sure there were going to be no other surprises inside me when they opened me up, they decided to do a MRI scan too. So the next day that was my trip out. A porter turned up with a wheelchair, and off we set, with a nurse 'just in case' coming along too.

On arrival I said to the nurse,
"I love this sort of treatment. You can do as many things as you like to me if you don't actually touch me!"
I liked this nurse, she often came to me on the ward. It's nice to have a friendly face with you. However, it turned out she wasn't allowed in the room with me. If you've never had an MRI scan, there's a list, quite a lengthy list, of people who can't have them. Because it is essentially a massive powerful magnet, anyone with any metal or machinery in them, can't have one. Got a pacemaker? Don't have an MRI, it can stop it working. Got a metal implant? Don't have an MRI, it'll rip it out through your skin (that must be impressive, if a little painful) as the magnet is that powerful. The nurse in question had a tattoo. Only a small one, but nevertheless a tattoo. And some inks contain metal.

I climbed out of the wheelchair and onto the scanner bed. They put a button in my hand; if I pressed it I could talk to them. The downside is, it stops the scan and anything done up to that point is lost. I was told the scan could take up to 40 minutes. The bed slid me, headfirst, into the scanner. I was to remain motionless at all times. A movement, any movement at all, would render the scan useless.

I was both surprised and alarmed at how long the scanner was. It seemed a never-ending tunnel. It was also surprisingly and alarmingly low. The ceiling was very close in on me, the walls were very close to my sides. I felt very trapped. Very, very trapped. Very, very, very trapped. Panic started to rise up inside me. I was consumed by rising panic and fear. The scanner whirred and clunked as it started scanning. This did nothing to calm me.

"Hold your breath for me," said a voice, barely audible over the machine.

"And breathe again."

About time too. My panic was hard enough to deal with without having a breathing competition going on too. All I could see was the confines of the scanner, very close to me on all sides. I shut my eyes. All I could hear was the scanner sounding even closer. There was no winning. I was hating it. I was in fear. I was panicking. I pressed the button.

"What is it?" said the voice.

"I'm sorry, I can't do it," I cried. I was sobbing now. "I thought I could. But I can't."

"It's ok," they said. But I knew it wasn't.

They got me out and sent me back to the ward. I really wasn't happy for the rest of the day. The fear and panic had won.

4 SEE YOU JIMMY

It's probably worth explaining at this point about my fear. For all my care-free approach and happy-go-lucky attitude, my Achilles heel is confined spaces and a feeling of being trapped.

When my middle child was born, (obviously they were the youngest at that point) they weren't very well. They spent the first three months of their life in an incubator on the neonatal ward. It had a Blue Peter badge on it. I was proud that all the milk bottle tops I had saved and all the stamps I had ripped carefully off letters as a child had been put to good use.

Although there were many issues for the doctors to deal with, and they did do admirably well, one condition required special-ist treatment at St James Hospital in Leeds, known to everyone as 'Jimmy's'.

Our brief was to arrive and check-in at the hospital for 10am. We'd never been to Leeds before in our lives, we didn't know how long it would take to get there, it was going to be rush hour too. We decided to go up the night before and stay in Leeds.

We set off and stopped at a McDonalds drive-through on the way. On arrival in Leeds, our plan was cunningly simple; stop at the first hotel we see, check-in and get them to give us a map or direc-tions to Jimmy's in the morning. After all, who is going to be stay-ing in Leeds on a cold, wet, weeknight in December?

It turns out everyone was staying in Leeds on a cold, wet, weeknight in December. The first hotel we saw was the Hilton, a massive skyscraper. They must have hundreds if not thousands of rooms.

"Sorry," said the receptionist when we asked about a room "We only have a suite left and that's £250 for the night. Room only."

You would think for £250 they could manage a bit of breakfast. Particularly bearing in mind it was 9pm and the room was otherwise going to be empty.

"Would you like me to ring round and see if anyone has vacancies?"

"Yes please."

And so it was that a few minutes later we were setting off for The Queens. Promised as being 'round the corner' they had promised us a room for the still ambitiously priced £75. But were prepared to throw in breakfast.

The Queens is a smart hotel. A very smart hotel. On arrival there's a man in a red frock coat who welcomes you as you pull up and, because guests staying there do nothing as vulgar as park their own car, takes your car keys and parks it for you. I was most embarrassed; we had two small children and the car was a tip, there were the remnants of the McDonald's too. He did it with good grace and didn't recoil when he got in, nor remove his red frock coat. Although I couldn't be sure, I'm fairly certain this was the first time in his job he'd driven a Skoda Felicia.

Again, the hotel didn't expect you to do anything as vulgar as find your own room, and you were escorted up there by the concierge. I now had two panics. One: we were going to use a lift, and two: were we expected to tip? And if so, how much? Okay, that's three panics.

I've never been a fan of lifts. I have a fear of being stuck in one. Some say this is an irrational fear, but it seems perfectly reasonable to me. However, I feel better if there's a member of staff in there too; if nothing else they will surely be missed and someone will search for them and discover a stuck lift. So we went up in the lift with the concierge. On arrival at the room he showed us in and around; presumably they must have people who don't know a bed and a TV and need these things pointing out. I was impressed that despite checking in only minutes ago, they already had a cot in the room. The concierge could clearly tell we weren't used to this sort of life, and left without even waiting for a tip.

The next morning there were no staff to take us down, so I used the stairs. On arrival at breakfast though, the hotel didn't expect you to do anything as vulgar as carry your own plate. So although it was a self-service buffet breakfast, someone in white gloves walked next to you carrying the plate. My arms felt like they'd just been made redundant.

Armed with clear directions to Jimmy's, we managed to get lost no more than six times. Maybe the concierge was holding a grudge about the tip as I'm perfectly capable of following decent directions.

I'm sure the people of Leeds can count perfectly well, but there's a rogue employee at Jimmy's who feels the traditional system of 1,2,3,4,etc is old-fashioned and out of date and they've come up with their own new system.

Walking in from ground level, where we parked the car, we checked where the ward was. Level 8. Ruth, who was then my wife and knew what I was thinking, gave me a look that said 'we are not walking up to the eighth floor, you can use a lift like everyone else.' And to be fair, she had a point. Or at least she would have had Leeds used numbers like everyone else.

Although I didn't know it then, it turns out that using the special Leeds numbering system, level 8 is actually the fifth floor. I'd walk to the fifth floor. In fact, I did thereafter.

It was a busy lobby on the ground floor-which turned out to be level 2-and there were four lifts. You pressed one button and a lift would appear. It took a while but a lift arrived. Everyone surged forward but as it was so busy we decided to wait.

Once the lift had gone, we pressed the button again. A hospital worker turned up with a trolley. A lift arrived and he got in with us. They only wanted one floor up, which from level 2 was naturally level 4. The lift stopped, the doors opened, he got out. The doors closed, the lift went. It was just us.

Suddenly the lift stopped. The doors didn't open. I panicked. I pressed the alarm button. Nothing. When I rule the world (and it's surely only a matter of time before I do), the first law I will pass is that when you're in a lift you can hear the alarm. You need the reassurance that at least it is working.

Of course, the trouble with panic is that all rational thinking deserts you. The trouble is you don't realise that, and you think you're the rational one. So, there we were stuck in a lift. Us two and a baby. I was pressing the alarm continually, partly out of panic and partly because I couldn't think of anything else to do.

Ruth tried to be calming
"At least we're altogether," she said.
"That's not a good thing, if one of us wasn't in here they could raise the alarm!" Why wasn't she being rational about this?
"It's only a lift, what's the worst that could happen?"
"WE COULD ALL DIE" I might have been a bit hysterical at this point.
"Why don't you sit on the floor and read your book?"
Read a book? At a time like this! That's like playing violins on the deck of the Titanic. But I couldn't come up with a better idea, so I sat down anyway and got my book out. But I couldn't concentrate on it. Not with impending death. If the lift didn't plummet to the floor, I wondered what we'd die of first; lack of oxygen or starvation and dehydration. The elephant in the room now was, who would we have to kill and eat first?
"Hello? Hello?" I was hearing voices now.
"Hello!" Ruth shouted back.

"Are you stuck?"

"Yes. We've got a baby, and my husband is...a bit...a bit...panicked!" Nicely understated.

"Don't worry, happens all the time," that's reassuring, "we will have you out in no time."

In fairness they had us out in no time. What had felt like a couple of weeks in the lift, turned out to be twenty minutes. As the lift doors opened on level 6, I shot out of the doors and up the stairs. It can't be an irrational fear if it actually happens can it?

5 GOING UNDER

They assured me it that it happened quite often that people didn't like MRI scans. But clearly not often enough for them to actually do anything about it.

Why not load you in feet first from the other end for example? Why not make the scanner a bit stronger so it could be further away from you? Apparently neither is an option. I knew this because I had a friend who worked as a radiologist and she came to visit me on her lunch breaks.

What they could do though, was give me medication to relax me. What they called 'happy pills.' Whenever a member of the hospital staff heard I was to be given these, they all said the same thing:
"You'll enjoy those."

I was given two to take an hour before my next MRI scan, and another on arrival at it. I didn't feel happy. I just felt sick. I said so. A cardboard bowl magically appeared. I was told because of the pills I could not drive or operate machinery. That was a relief, I'd been worried I'd have to operate the scanner. Now I had an excuse to say no if they asked me to.

To help relax I could choose a CD to listen to. They had a choice of two. Both were free with a Sunday paper. One was 'Classical' the other 'Easy listening.' I went for 'Easy Listening. '

They spent some time with me, showing me round the machine.

They let me peer through it. Then it was time to get in. This time I was joined by the cardboard bowl, because I'd been worried there was too much space in there last time, best fill it up. I regretted saying I felt sick. One of the team stayed with my legs, the other went to the head end to show me how close to the end my head really was. And how much better it would have been to go in feet first from that end.

I can't say I felt relaxed or happy. The overwhelming feeling was sick. But I guess that's progress from fear. I did, with the help of The Sunday Times CD called, at a guess, "Songs you hoped you'd never hear again," get through it though. So I guess the pills worked in some way. The CD was hard listening though.

After all the tests and all the results had come through, it was confirmed I was to have a quintuple bypass. This resulted in my having to be moved to the cardiac surgical ward. The surgical ward was kept sterile. This made it sound like the other wards were on the grubby side.

Each day a cleaner would come into my room and brush and mop. Once a week was a big clean. This was the same but involved moving furniture. As there really isn't anywhere much to move a hospital bed in a hospital room, and I wasn't allowed to get out of the bed, the solution was to raise the bed to its fullest height so they could clean under it.

It felt strange being on a bed so close to the ceiling, but the cleaner chatted away underneath, and I was soon brought down again. The days continued in the same routine.

They came to move me just as I was finishing lunch. When I got to the new ward they were just about to start serving lunch, so I had another one. I do like my food.

In my new ward, I got a bed in a ward of six. Three of the other occupants were in their seventies. The fourth was 92, and the fifth was originally from Birmingham but now lived in Thailand. One of the men in their seventies cut himself each morning trying to shave with the NHS issue disposable razors. The man from Thailand was itching to get back there and wanted to know when he'd be able to fly again after the operation. It wasn't good news for him. A spring in Birmingham hadn't been on his plan.

The days rolled by and we had got to Christmas Eve by the time my operation was confirmed. I've had better Christmas presents. They couldn't fit me in on Christmas Eve, so I was going to be the day after Boxing Day. I had two days to contemplate my fate.

It felt a bit unfair to be delayed two days because of Christmas. But when I mentioned this to the consultant he said,
"It's better than being so ill we need to operate on you on Christmas Day."
He'd got a point.

Waking up on Christmas morning in hospital does lack the excitement of waking up on Christmas morning at home. But they do try. The nurses all wore a Christmas jumper and we had a present each. The man across from me had been given a shaving gift set, and because I was going to be allowed out of bed to shower, I was given a shower gel gift set. We were all chuffed to bits. The Brummie was given a travel wash bag, which seemed a little insensitive.

They serve a full Christmas lunch. They even add a Christmas cracker to your tray. We were allowed out of bed to the day room to watch the Queens speech on the telly. It was probably as well we all had visitors in the afternoon or we might even have played charades.

In true Christmas Day style, we had a buffet tea, but less traditionally served on a trolley wheeled onto the ward. But we were allowed out of bed to help ourselves.

Boxing Day was back to business as usual pretty much, although no tests or procedures took place. Kristyan and Becky came over in the evening with a couple of other friends and we had our own party. They brought crackers and games.

At bedtime I was told my last meal (I'm sure they didn't really mean last, did they?) would be twelve hours before my operation. I was to be at one in the afternoon. So they would wake me at one in the morning with coffee and toast.

Reassuringly they woke up the wrong person. The Brummie wasn't too happy at being woken. They then came to wake me with tea and toast by mistake. I don't even drink tea. This wasn't going at all well.

When you come out of the operation, rather than going back onto the ward, you go into Intensive Care so the ward want all your belongings taken away. Mum came to take my bag of stuff and say goodbye. A last meal and a final farewell. They know how to cheer you up.

It's hard not to feel melancholy at moments like this, so fortunately a friend who is a nurse popped in to see me on her break, which cheered me up no end. Then they came to take me away.

I was wheeled down in my bed to the theatre. You are then transferred from the ward bed to a theatre bed. Normally an easy process, but my bed would not adjust to the same height as the theatre bed. After a lot of scratching of heads, it was decided they would use the board.

I didn't like the sound of the board. It sounded more like an instrument of torture than an aid. I offered just to move over but they seemed excited to use the board as they don't normally get to use it.

Basically, they slid a board under me, then having gathered together quite a few staff, man-handled me over to the other bed, then removed the board like a magician. Only I wasn't levitating, I was just on the adjacent bed.

I was then put in a waiting area. Someone came to check I was me and what I was in for. They then removed my notes and replaced them with a 42. I was no longer a free man, but a number.

Two porters came to collect 42 and I was wheeled through to the room before the theatre. I didn't want to ever see the theatre. If I saw the theatre, something had gone badly wrong.

My arm was stretched out and twisted into an uncomfortable position. Two doctors then spent some time inserting needles into my arm. Then a nice man with a friendly face said,
"OK, I'm going to put you to sleep now. I want you to count to 10 for me."
I guess it was too late to ask for someone who knew how to count.
"1, 2, 3, 4."
I was unconscious.

6 A WALK IN THE PARK

I awoke confused. There was a tube in my mouth down my throat. They'd told me about this, but it didn't make it any more pleasant to wake up to. Obviously they knew it was there, and that they were waking me up, so they knew to take it out. But I felt the need to remind them anyway. I couldn't talk with the tube in, so just grunted, pointed to the tube and mimed pulling it out.

"It's okay," said a nurse I couldn't see.

She removed the tube. I looked down at my body. Where once my fine manly chest had been (it's my story, I can tell it how I like) there was now a big dressing and a lot of blood. The heart monitor was still attached and there were three tubes disappearing into my stomach area.

"I will take the tubes out now," said the nurse.

But I was too confused still.

"What time is it?" I asked.

"It's 2 o'clock," said the nurse. My confused brain accepted that for a minute before realising that made nothing any clearer.

"2 o'clock when?" I asked.

"Saturday morning."

I'd been under for thirteen hours.

They pulled the tubes out one by one. It hurt a lot. They told me to breathe in whilst they did it. I think that was to stop me screaming. I had a quick look over my body to see if anything else was still waiting to be taken out and even more importantly if it looked like it would hurt. The only thing was a catheter. I'd never had one before, but at least it meant I didn't need to get up for the toilet.

I'd had an anaesthetic three times before in my life. On each occasion I was very sick afterwards. I felt sick now but couldn't decide if what I felt most was sick or in pain.

"What do you want to eat?" said a nurse who was far too cheerful. "Nothing. I feel sick." A cardboard bowl appeared from some disembodied hands behind me.
"Wrong answer!" said the annoyingly cheerful nurse. "Toast? Yogurt?"
"Okay," I was beaten into submission by happiness, "I'll have a yogurt."
"Right answer." He produced a strawberry yogurt.
I ate half of it and was promptly sick. It filled the cardboard bowl and more. Nurses came and mopped up and got me a new cardboard bowl.
"Told you I didn't want to eat."
"You won't get better and can't go home till you've eaten."
Undeniably true, but having had my chest ripped open and my breastbone sawn through, being sick really didn't make me feel better either.

The day passed with me mainly dozing in and out of consciousness. My mum came to see me, I don't think I was much company, but I appreciated it nevertheless. A friend who was a church minister turned up next. He was wearing his dog collar. Visiting in Intensive Care is limited to close relations. A dog collar acts as an 'Access All Areas' pass.
"How is it?" he asked. "A walk in the park?"
I'd just been sick and my stomach was keen to go again. Being sick isn't usually pleasant, but when you can't move and just sitting is painful and retching pulls on your chest stitches, it's even less fun.
"Yeah, a walk in the park. In Beirut. With snipers aiming at you."
I was sick again.

I had some toast and wasn't sick for at least a minute, so they seized the opportunity and took me back to a ward. Intensive Care is very clinical, the ward was a more relaxing atmosphere. I was put into a bay of six, in the far corner by the window. Not that there was much of a view. But it didn't matter I wasn't in much of a position to appreciate it. I told them I felt ill. They said everyone in hospital does.

Lots of people came to see me and I appreciated them all, but I really don't think I was much company. Sometimes I'd be asleep and wake up to find a friend standing there. They were never sure whether to wake me or not. I was never sure how long they'd been standing there watching me sleep. I was still feeling quite ill. I'd now quite happily stay in bed, but having confined me to it for two weeks, they were now obsessed with getting me out of it. I told them I was feeling ill. You'll feel better for getting up they said. I didn't.

One evening I was heading at a snail pace to the bathroom, when diarrhoea struck. It came on with no warning, and I couldn't do much else but stand there. To anyone watching me, they'd be hard pressed to notice the difference between my walking speed and stationary. But the diarrhoea was harder to hide. Nurse call bells were pressed and the nurses duly arrived. I was assisted to the bathroom, stripped off, wiped down and showered. All without any of it involving any input from me.

I was taken back to bed. Where I promptly had diarrhoea again. I'd told them I was ill.

They repeated the bathroom procedure. I don't care how much these people are paid, it's not enough to deal with that. This time when I came out, I was put into a single room. The fear was, if I had an infection they didn't want me giving it to everybody else. I felt much better now though, but I thought I might sound unappreciative if I mentioned it.

To perform a heart bypass they create a new artery around the blockage, thus creating a bypass. They obviously need to access your heart to do this, but your health and recovery is improved if they do this without stopping your heart. How they do this I can't begin to imagine. But they did.

The new arteries they created were formed from veins taken from my leg. Think about that for a moment. How does that even work? My schoolboy understanding of biology meant I understood my heart pumped blood round my body in arteries and veins. One taking it from the heart, the other returning it. On this basis all arteries must become veins at some point on their journey round the body. If they've removed a vein from my leg, what happens to the blood in the artery? Why isn't my leg full of loose blood? Maybe they block the whole artery, but then my leg would have no blood. I just had to hope they knew what they were doing.

Each morning two physiotherapists would arrive on the ward and take us for exercise. Partly to get our hearts going, partly to exercise our legs with veins missing. The first few days just a walk to the ward day room and back was more than enough. But gradually the trips grew longer. Finally, the day came to go off the ward.

The next day was the day to tackle stairs. Just up one flight, a sit down, then back down. Complete that and you got the red stairs badge. Get the gold marathon badge and you could go home. Without the gold badge you had to stay in hospital.

To get the gold badge you had to walk out of the ward, along a corridor, up the stairs, along a corridor, back down some more stairs, along a corridor and back to the ward. Not a vast distance and less than my visitors were doing to come and see me. But then they hadn't had heart surgery.

I got my gold on the first attempt. It was the proudest achievement of my life. I was a free man.

Each day my dressings on my chest were changed and a new surgical stocking put on my vein-less leg. The dressing changing wasn't too bad. The stocking changing was a skilled art. The stockings were, it appeared, three sizes too small. However, the point was to keep it tight on my leg so my leg didn't swell, presumably from all the loose blood sloshing around down there. Some nurses were much better at this than others.

It takes a long time to get discharged from hospital. In the morning the doctor says you can go home. Everyone is happy for you to go home. The only thing stopping you is the medication you require. This is medication you've had every day whilst you've been in hospital, so they clearly have plenty. It's medication you can get from any pharmacy, with a prescription, at a moments notice. Yet, it takes a hospital all day to get it.

My sister came to pick me up at lunchtime. But I didn't have any clothes so she went to get some. She went to collect her son from school. She had tea. Finally, she came back for me. I was still waiting for the medication.

Eventually it turned up. They said,
"You'll need to take these for the rest of your life. Here's two weeks supply." Clearly they weren't confident.
And with that, I was sent out into the big, wide world after three weeks of being in hospital. My sister pushed me, in a hospital wheelchair, to the entrance. Where she left me while she went to bring her car closer. Her son said,
"What if someone steals him whilst we are gone?"
"They'll soon bring him back!"
My sister loves me really.

The first week out, I went home and my other sister stayed with me. The problem you don't realise in hospital is how everything is designed to help. My settee at home is very comfy and I normally have no problem getting down to it and up off it. But recovering from a major operation, I found it too low and too deep to sit on.

My stairs were suddenly incredibly steep. My bed was suddenly woefully inadequate without a remote control to adjust my position. Indeed, I found it impossible to sit up, or get up, without assistance. We purchased a thing so I could go to the toilet in the night without the need to get up. Modern technology at its best.

The district nurse came to visit and change my dressings. And left a supply of surgical stockings for my leg. These were so tight as to be virtually impossible to put on. It often took my sister the best part of the day to change them.

7 ENTERING REHAB

The physiotherapist's instructions, when I left hospital, were clear; go for a walk three days a week. 5 minutes in the first week. 10 minutes in the second week. 15 minutes in the third and 20 in the fourth. It seemed an impossible goal when it took me nearly half an hour just to get to the bathroom. But I did it.

When I did my first walk from home, my family were all round so came too. A simple, very easy 'round the block' walk. With hindsight this was probably over ambitious. Although it's really no distance, and up until that point I'd never even noticed it was uphill, it took over the allotted 5 minutes. My sister-in-law even offered to get her car half-way round, which seemed pointless as I could see it, but it took several minutes to get there. My nieces lapped me. Twice. But I did it. I did it twice more that week too and got faster each time.

The next week my sister had to return home, so I went to stay with my mum. It is what mums are for. I mean, at our ages the care is usually the other way around, but still.

My walks went further, but fortunately where Mum lives is perfectly flat. We ventured to the post box. On one ambitious trip we went to visit an old family friend who I knew lived close by. It had never taken so long to get there before. We had a rest and a drink there before the slow walk back.

And so the walks grew. Thankfully, despite it being January, the weather wasn't too bad. I gradually improved, but I could still feel my breastbone rubbing together where it had been broken, as it healed back together. I wasn't allowed to lift or carry.

One afternoon I felt quite ill and went really cold. Mum got me another jumper. I was still cold. She got me a duvet, and I sat there wrapped up. At teatime I was feeling better and went into the kitchen to eat tea with Mum. Of course, by then I was feeling too hot, so had to open the back door to let the freezing January air in. Mum had to sit there in the cold whilst I sweated it out. It is what parents do for their children.

But generally I was, slowly but surely, getting better day by day.

Eventually my walking had improved to such an extent that I was ready to head to the shops. Mum and I set off and headed to Sainsbury's. A mile there and, not unsurprisingly, a mile back. My longest walk so far. I did feel very conscious, as by now my walking speed was up to normal, that to everyone who saw us, I looked like a fit and healthy man letting an elderly woman carry two bags of hefty shopping whilst I swanned next to her empty handed. The reality was she was far healthier and in better shape than me. It just shows how much appearances can be deceptive.

The British Heart Foundation (BHF) have a booklet guiding you through recovery. According to that, after four weeks I could do some light dusting. So there was something to look forward to. Although I couldn't work out what would be deemed heavy dusting. The week after that I could prepare simple light meals. But as I couldn't lift a kettle or saucepan it did seem to limit it to micro-wave meals.

My recovery progressed. I started going out on the bus; I couldn't drive for three months and was off work for six months. Buses are ideal if you want to go where they go, when they go. My choice of destinations was limited, particularly as I had to be back for the last bus to Mum's house, which was a very late two o'clock in the afternoon! I'm sure more people would travel by bus if the timetable suited the passengers not the bus operators. But public transport has never been hot on customer service.

Then the letter came from the hospital. I could start the rehabilitation programme. I was invited to a check-over at the hospital and then the BHF would meet me at the gym and guide me through a rehab program. I'd never been to a gym in my life.

I'd always thought gyms were a bit pointless. If people cycled or ran to the gym instead of driving, they wouldn't need to go to the gym. Let's be honest, I was also a bit scared it would be full of big butch muscular figures, making me feel even more inadequate.

All the rehab heart patients turned up. We met in a small room first of all and the BHF team took our blood pressure and pulses. We then went out into the gym. We had one to one instruction, and they started us off gently. I had a go on the treadmill and a bike. I was surprised how much I enjoyed myself.

The next week they threw a rowing machine and a cross trainer into the mix. Each week they added more, each week they made me work harder and longer on each one. Don't get me wrong, I was still doing very little compared to the regular gym people, but I was doing more each week and that's all that mattered.

After several weeks of going every Wednesday with the BHF rehab team, I was allowed to start going for a couple of extra sessions each week on my own. This was all free and funded by the NHS and BHF as part of the treatment. I felt I owed it to the NHS to look after myself given what it must have cost to keep me in hospital for three weeks and the operation too. Equally, I had no intention of going through that again.

Despite my previous lack of gym experience, indeed verging on phobia, I was actually really enjoying it. When I got to the end of the rehab sessions, I even signed up for more. They had a deal with the gym, three months for just £12. That's £1 a week. I'm not one to turn down a bargain.

However, gym membership isn't cheap. So at the end of that offer, however much I had enjoyed myself, I wasn't going to pay for more and my gym life ended as abruptly as it had begun. My rehab was now down to me and me alone.

Walking, and running, are healthy, good for you and most importantly free. So I decided that's what I'd do. It was time to find some walks and put on the walking shoes.

8 SOUTH WEST ADVENTURES

I was very fortunate at this time to be working in Devon. Plenty of walking opportunities. I even, for one brief moment, had a mad plan to walk the whole South West Coast Path. At 630 miles it stretches from Minehead to Poole. But I soon realised this would be a massive undertaking. To be honest not so much the walking, but either carrying a tent and equipment round me with, or ridiculously expensive stopping in hotels or B&Bs each night. Instead I did a few short sections, easy day walks.

The first thing I noticed on my first foray onto the coast path is that you can't often actually see the coast. You're tantalisingly close, but often a massive hedgerow grows between you and it, blocking the view. The other thing I quickly found was that the coast isn't flat. Okay, strictly speaking the coast is flat, it's just the route the path takes isn't flat. There's a surprising number of cliffs in Devon. Cliffs may occasionally involve a downhill, but certainly they involve an uphill.

My first adventure started in the seaside town of Exmouth. The path casually dumps its walkers there on the bank of the river Exe, as the walk continues on the opposite bank at Dawlish Warren. Making your way between the two is your problem. It's not far as the crow flies. Not far at all. But due to the lack of a bridge it's a long detour inland, or needs a boat.

I started in Exmouth and walked along its pleasant sea front. At the end of this there's a footpath zigzagging its way up the cliff. Fortunately, before you start the climb there's an ice cream kiosk, so it seemed wise to stock up on calories for the climb ahead.

I arrived at the top of the cliff and was rewarded with a view over Exmouth and beyond to Dawlish. Thoughtful benches were provided to sit and admire the view, so I did.

Admiring views is very nice but doesn't get the mileage done. So I got up, and carried on. The beauty of the South West Coast Path, is that it's, mainly at least, clear where to go. The path is well worn and well marked. If you can tell the difference between path, and not a path, you can't go wrong.

Despite being on top of the cliff, once I set off the path rose still higher. The cliffs at this point are made of a distinctive red sandstone. It's very pretty from the beach. But when you're stood on top of it, it really could be made of anything.

The problem with sandstone is that it's not very structurally sound. Large parts of the cliff crumble down into the sea with brutal regularity round here. It's best not to stand too close to the edge, otherwise you may unintentionally end up on the beach below.

I hurried on. Round a few headlands and around three miles later I came to a caravan holiday park. The fact this holiday park was so huge, yet hadn't been visible till I was virtually at it, is testament to its design. A massive holiday park, literally thousands of caravans, made totally invisible by the landscape.

The coastal path skirts the edge of the park, but the park runs down to the beach, so it's impossible not to enter the park. I'm guessing you're allowed to follow the path and not venture into the complex. But then again they did have an ice cream kiosk and a shop not far off the path; surely they wouldn't deny me spending money with them.

As it turned out, I didn't spend any money in the shop. I had to pass their onsite restaurant on the way to the shop and I hadn't had lunch, so dropped in there instead. Eating alone on a family holiday park I did feel conspicuous, but no one batted an eyelid.

After a lovely lunch, which was far better than I was expecting from a holiday park family restaurant, I carried on. But not far. Something caught my eye. It was a bus stop. The bus stop had a picture of an open-top bus on it. I'm a sucker for an open-top bus. A quick look at the timetable revealed I had forty minutes to kill. No problem, I'd have a quick look to see where the path went, then be back for the bus. The thought of retracing my steps all the way to Exmouth had never really appealed, but there was no obvious circular walk.

The path continued through the car park and round the outer perimeter of the holiday park. Only now, with the holiday park on my left, the sea on my right had been replaced by a military firing range. Gunshots rang out. It must be quite relaxing for the holidaymakers to hear gunshots. The path climbed steeply, then bore round to the left to what clearly had been a path down to another beach. It was now fenced off, the sandy beach below no longer accessible. The cliff had crumbled and a large section of it sat on the beach to serve as a reminder of the danger.

The clifftop footpath carried on to Budleigh Salterton, which the signpost promised was five miles away, but with no direct bus back, and only a limited bus service to anywhere. I turned round.

I headed back to the bus stop. The open-top bus duly trundled into view and came to a wheezing stop. It was the end of its route and it had a few minutes to wait before heading back to Exmouth.

I got on and there was a very jolly friendly lady driver. I went, of course, upstairs. People who sit downstairs on double deckers for no good reason worry me. People who sit downstairs on open-top double deckers worry me even more.

The bus set off. It headed uphill through the maze of caravans. They stretched even further inland than I'd first realised, and we really had climbed quite a bit. I don't think you could honestly say these caravans were walkable from the beach. The bus then set off into town. I love being able to peer over fences and walls and look into otherwise off-limits views.

On an open-too bus, you also get the added thrill of being hit in the face by a low hanging branch. It's all part of the fun.

My next trip on the South West Coast path started across the Exe at Dawlish Warren. The Warren is basically a large sand spit formed from the sand of Dawlish getting washed up by the tide. The distance across the Exe mouth to Exmouth isn't that great, and is slowly closing.

Were it not for the river you could easily walk from Dawlish Warren to Exmouth. But with the river you'd get wet feet. And head. There are also really strong undercurrents. All things considered, it's best to get a boat across.

There are two boats from Exmouth. One is rather expensive but more substantial and sails to Starcross. The other is a cheaper but considerably smaller water taxi to Dawlish Warren. Or you can skirt round the river Exe inland on the much longer but considerably cheaper train or bus.

For those of us who live inland, there is something a bit special about getting a boat. This is the stuff of holidays. It's something different. Of course, the boat companies know this and therefore charge a premium for it in the hope holidaymakers just pay up.

The true test of value for money is how many locals use it. I couldn't see anyone who didn't look touristy. There weren't any Devonian accents. Clearly the locals didn't use this. Then again, it went to Starcross. No offence to Starcross residents but there isn't really anything to go to Starcross for. Except the novelty of the post office being in the pub.

I imagine many a Starcross man tells his wife each evening he's got a letter to post. It's certainly an imaginative way to keep a post office open.

The reason the ferry sails to Starcross is historical. It's the railways. You know this because the ferry departure point can only be reached from the station platform. In times gone by, train tickets to Exmouth could be used to Starcross and the ferry across. They can't now, that's progress for you.

To say Starcross is a hamlet is to talk it up. But the main A379 thunders through with the Exe, railway and road all cosily together. There's a pub which doubles as the post office, a small shop, a sailing club and a golf club. Along with the station and ferry that's pretty much it. There is a chip shop too, but it was shut when I was there.

It's not unpretty though. There are thatched cottages and pretty gardens. There's also a building whose front door pillars actually stick out onto the A379. It's listed so can't be moved, but they certainly don't use that door anymore. Every summer there are bottlenecks here as holidaymakers try to manoeuvre their caravans around it.

Of course from here you need to walk, or get a bus or train to Dawlish Warren. It's quite a detour just to get across a river. I walked, I was here to walk anyway and it was a lovely summers day. I went down the road, it is right next to the railway line. There's a fence between you and the track, but the trains come fast enough and close enough to startle you each time. It doesn't take long to clear Starcross and the road then goes alongside the golf course before arriving in Cockwood.

There's a small harbour in Cockwood, from which you can't see the sea. The railway line blocks the view, running as it does, between the harbour and the river. Can you imagine the uproar these days if you wanted to build that? There are two small bridges so boats can get in and out, but only the smallest of boats can access it.

The main road bends away inland at this point but I took the minor road round through Cockwood. Initially following the road, the path then tucks into land between the railway and road, before emerging at the road and crossing over it, to do the same on the other side.

It does make walking much more pleasant not being right next to the traffic. As the path approaches Dawlish Warren, it's back to the road to make way for the holiday parks. "Bingo every night" boasts one, "Stay here 50 weeks of the year" brags another. One has an on-site pharmacy which doesn't bode well. How do you even sustain an injury playing bingo?

You come to a mini roundabout. To the left, a low bridge takes you under the railway to the beach. To the right, the road wends uphill back to join the main road you left behind in Cockwood. Although you can walk along the sea front from here all the way to Dawlish, walking between the sea and the railway, the coastal path takes a different route.

I turned right, as if to follow the road uphill, but just before "Lee's Bar" the footpath disappears into the woods. Lee's Bar has a sign outside advertising "Free beer tomorrow for those that missed it yesterday." Lee clearly has a sense of humour.

The path then turns off the road and starts heading uphill. It takes you behind the Langstone Cliff hotel, and you get to peek in the grounds and see the outdoor swimming pool as you pass. There were plenty of people in it when I passed, making the most of the sun.

The path continues uphill and would offer spectacular views if the hedge was lower on the sea side. But instead all you can see are brambles and hedges. The path levels out at the top and signs of life emerge, as house rooftops appear over the hedges.

The path eventually dumps you out on the road, which you can follow all the way into Dawlish. Or you can turn off again part way down, use a bridge to cross the railway, and walk the path you left at The Warren between the sea and the railway.

For most of its way the path runs at the same height as the railway, but coming into Dawlish it drops to sea level, making the path inaccessible at low tide. The reason for this is that at this point there are houses on the other side of the railway line. When the the line was built, the house owners didn't want working class people walking along the sea front to see into their houses so the path dropped below the railway line.

The sea wall is therefore narrower at this point. This was the place where the storm of February 2014 breached the wall. The waves had been battering the wall all day but into the evening the storm grew even stronger and smashed through the wall, washing away everything under the track and leaving the line suspended over nothing.

Train services were suspended till repairs were completed in the April, and to try to prevent it happening again the wall was made full thickness and the path brought up to rail height. But you still can't see into the houses, not without binoculars anyway.

The path continues into Dawlish, passing the station, the platform of which overhangs the beach. The coastal path carries on up Lea Mount. But the sea wall path continues on around the bottom of the mount to what is now called Coryton Cove, formally known as the Gentleman's Bathing Beach. In the Victorian era people of different genders couldn't be seen to be mixing together in a state of undress. Even if the undress was a neck to knee bathing costume.

There are several paths up Lea Mount and the road goes up the side of it too. The paths criss-cross to the top, zig-zagging in a failed attempt to lessen the slope. There are lots of seats and shelters on the way up (or on the way down, paths are very flexible like that.) You can stop to catch your breath or just to admire the views, which really are quite stunning. The railway, of course, tunnels through its base.

When you get to the top, there's a nice grassy area and it's peaceful and tranquil. You'd never know there was an A Road next to you on one side, a railway main line below you and the untamed sea on the other side.

The path continues out onto the road and follows it for a while, before disappearing off down a field to the sea. The path slopes downhill to the railway line and you lose all the height you gained going up Lea Mount. It follows the railway for a short distance before veering back inland and back uphill. You trudge back uphill to emerge back on the road just a few yards further down from where the path left the road to head to the sea. It really is the most pointless bit of path. You feel its only purpose is so they can say the path follows the coast whenever possible. But it's a lengthy hilly detour for no real need.

It's the road's turn now to go downhill. Something it does all the way into Teignmouth. However, the path veers off again down a pleasant sideroad and makes its way to the railway, which has been clinging to the sea all the way from Dawlish Warren. Here, there's a pedestrian tunnel under the railway and the path resumes its place between the sea and rail to Teignmouth.

Teignmouth is a pleasant town with a selection of shops and cafes, a pier, crazy golf; everything you could ask of a seaside town really. It also has a street called 'The street with no name' which really is an excellent name for a street, if a little self-defeating. They even made a street sign with it on. A true oxymoron.

Not unsurprisingly, the river Teign has its mouth here. This creates a second beach behind the main one. What the locals call the back beach. There's a ferry service from here over the river to Shaldon.

Shaldon is a quintessential English town. There's a pub, church and village green. Everyone knows everyone. And everyone knows about everyone. It's just that they also have a small zoo and a smugglers tunnel. Few English villages can boast those.

The smugglers tunnel is surprisingly long, and takes you under the cliff to a beach that can't be accessed any other way, apart from the sea obviously. Thus it was ideal for smuggling. I'm assuming back then, the tunnel was neither lit, nor signposted 'smugglers tunnel leading to smugglers beach.' There probably wasn't deckchair hire either.

If it had been signposted, the job of the customs men would have been much easier. These days, of course, the good people of Shaldon don't do smuggling any more. Or at least I couldn't find any who'd admit to it. Mind you, they are still adept at taking a lot of money off you. Just try asking for an ice cream or an admission ticket for the zoo.

I followed the SouthWest Coast Path up a steep hill in woodland on top of the smugglers tunnel, but I could have been anywhere and there were no views to be had.

The coastal path carries ever onward on its six hundred and thirty-mile journey. But for me it was time to head home.

9 A SPARE CATHEDRAL

There is a song that scousers sing with pride, the chorus of which goes:

In my Liverpool home, La-de-da,
In my Liverpool home.
We speak with an accent exceedingly rare,
We meet under a statue exceedingly bare,
If you want a cathedral, we've got one to spare,
In my Liverpool home.

My partner, Cath, had brought me to Liverpool for a day out. I had been before, but not for a long time, and we'd never been there together. We'd gone by train and we emerged from Lime Street station into the thronging city centre.

There's a tricky road junction to navigate and although there are traffic lights and pedestrian crossings, none of them in any way seem coordinated. So you have to wait on each traffic island for each set of traffic lights to change several times, before you can get across the road. Then repeat this several times for each road. It's not a great welcome.

We walked down to the main shopping centre, called Liverpool ONE. In there, both the local football teams have a shop. Everton called theirs the simply brilliant name 'Everton Two.' Which, of course, makes their postal address: Everton Two, Liverpool ONE.

However, we weren't here to shop, we were here for sport. Also in Liverpool ONE is an indoor crazy golf course. You may be about to try and argue that crazy golf is not a sport, but I say if we live in a world where snooker and darts are sports, then crazy golf must be a sport too.

It was February so we were glad it was indoors, indeed we had shunned outdoor courses for this reason. We played our 18 holes and despite the exertion of playing sport, I can't say my heartbeat was racing. So we went for a walk.

We walked through the city and down to the river. The former dock area has now been transformed into a tourist trap. Shops, bars and museums abound. A couple of which make no claims to have anything to do with the Beatles. There seems no limit to the amount the city is willing to cash in on the Fab Four.

We sat on the riverside to eat our packed lunch, shunning the offer to dine in a Yellow Submarine on Penny Lane owned by Eleanor Rigby. It really was very windy and although sitting by water is always preferable to sitting by a road, the view wasn't that stunning.

The Mersey was a dirty grey colour, reflecting the dirty grey colour of the sky. Across the Mersey was the town of Birkenhead. From our bench it too looked a dirty grey, but it must have greenery as it is home to the world's first publicly funded park. It opened in 1847 and is now a Grade 1 listed landscape. But it doesn't have a crazy golf course so I couldn't think of a reason to visit.

Towering upwards in Birkenhead, we could also see the ventilation shafts at the entrance to the Mersey Tunnel. It's not, naturally enough, open to pedestrians and we didn't have a car. I had been through it before on a bus; it's everything you expect of a tunnel, and not that exciting. I just remember it being longer than I'd thought it would be.

On the opposite bank of the Mersey to our draughty seat, was a cruise liner docked at Birkenhead ship works. The Cammell Laird works covers an impressive 130 acres and has been open since

1828. You can see why the people of Birkenhead wanted a park though. Impressive the ship works may be, attractive they are not.

Lunch finished, we set off to walk to the cathedrals. Starting out on a level walk down the road, we ended up cutting through a housing estate. Walking down one road, the trees all had hand knitted scarves on. There was nothing to explain this phenomenon. I doubt the trees of Liverpool feel the cold more than any others though.

We carried on to find ourselves looking up at the Anglican cathedral. Although not a particularly tall hill, it is on top of a hill, and from where we were standing, a steep hill.

We battled on. The entrance was, of course, on the furthest side from us. We went in from the cold, puffing and panting. Although a traditional and old-looking building, the cathedral is actually quite modern. The foundation stone was laid in 1904 and it was officially completed in 1978. To be fair, they had had two World Wars to contend with too.

Being modern, it doesn't have all the old plaques and tombs you usually get in a cathedral. Yet it doesn't seem to benefit from cheaper costs either. They currently have an appeal to raise 24 million pounds. It is a nice building though and personally, one of my favourite cathedrals. If you're allowed to have favourite cathedrals.

We carried on across the city to the Catholic cathedral. This is a much more modern looking building. Work started in 1962 and it was consecrated in 1967. Mind you, there were no World Wars to contend with in this time.

In fairness, the Catholic cathedral is smaller than its Anglican rival. But it's still the largest Catholic cathedral in the UK. It stands high on a hill at which we arrived at the bottom. A seemingly never-ending staircase led up to it. Possibly a stairway to heaven. Maybe that was their thought. No worries though if you can't make the stairs, they've thoughtfully provided a gift shop at the bottom. You can stock up on cathedral pencils and tea towels without actually needing to go in the cathedral itself.

The main round building rises upwards with the sides being formed of stained glass. It's a most impressive effect inside. Outside, like many buildings of the 1960s, it's mostly concrete. Also, like many 1960s buildings and other hastily constructed buildings, it had a few structural problems. Most notably leaks. It was extensively refurbished in the 1990s as a result.

We headed back to the station. We'd completed several miles walking. You often forget that city walking is walking, as you're usually aiming to get somewhere, rather than just being there for the walk. You overlook the mileage involved to get there, and back.

We'd had an enjoyable day out, we'd played crazy golf, we'd seen a stretch of water, we'd been in two cathedrals and we'd walked several miles. What more do you want from a day out?

10 THE LURE OF
THE SEA

Cath and I both love the sea. It's possibly because we live so far inland that it seems much more appealing. Instead of being surrounded by a cityscape, you can stand on the beach and look out at a vast open nothingness. And wind turbines. And the odd boat. But mainly nothingness.

The other beauty of the sea is there's always somewhere to walk. It's good for the souls. We set off for North Wales and a coastal stroll.

There are a number of seaside resorts in North Wales. The first one you come to is Prestatyn. We headed to the beach but just before we got there, we came to a crazy golf course. It would be rude not to play a round. Nine holes successfully putted, we carried on to the beach.

Keeping the sea to our right, we followed the path stretching off all the way to Rhyl. After clearing Prestatyn, there's a public information board telling you the delights of Prestatyn and Rhyl and that the promenade stretches between the two. That's the sort of exercise we like-promenade stretches.

We carried on. A lot of the path was covered in sand blown up off the beach. There were rows of wind turbines far out in the sea, most spinning round, but an odd rogue one resolutely not turning. Maybe they'd blown all the sand onto the path; they were pointing inland after all.

We passed a golf course on the land side. How anyone can play golf with such a wind blowing in off the sea I have no idea. Ironically, to me golf is crazy. Crazy golf, conversely, is perfectly normal. Hitting a ball across an open field seems mad-or crazy. Hitting a ball through obstacles and missing rotating windmill blades, seems a perfectly reasonable game of skill.

I don't know how many holiday caravans there are in Prestatyn and Rhyl, but from where we stood now, I'd guess somewhere in the low zillions. They stretch as far as you can see in all directions-well not out to sea obviously- different holiday parks merging endlessly into one.

There were then some bungalows, yards from the sea, and all perfectly positioned to get no view of it at all. After that were some modern flats, or apartments as they'd probably rather call them, all positioned to get a view of the sea. They were also inside an enclosed gated area with "Keep out. Private property" signs everywhere. They might have the view, but I bet they have less friends.

The path goes round a headland and Rhyl comes into view. From a distance, it could be any seaside town. There is a tower rising to the sky and a clutch of buildings on the sea front.

As you get closer, you see the plans were great, but overly ambitious. There's a large paved area which gives the appearance of being a performance area, or a stage for outdoor events. It was deserted. There was a brick building with a picture of a train on the roof but the shutters were all down. Out of one shutter, the brick paving had been laid to look like a train track. Clearly this had been a road train at one point. The rust on the shutters and the sand blown up against them suggested it hadn't run in many years. That, and the fact it was a hot sunny day and there was no sign of life.

We walked on. They really have made the area next to the beach quite pleasant. But there were very few people there. We came across a small fun fair. Small being the word. But, it did also have a crazy golf course with a welsh theme too. We were the only people on the course. It took us a while to locate the person to get the clubs and balls from. They clearly hadn't expected any customers to turn up.

Another victory in the bag, we continued down the front, passing another crazy golf course on the way. We strolled onto the beach and felt the sand between our toes. We jumped waves with our trousers rolled up. At the end of Rhyl sea front, the River Clwyd flows into the sea and this forms a natural, if abrupt, end to the walk. But turn inland and you find Marine Lake.

To walk around Marine Lake is around a mile, and isn't unpleasant. There is grass on three sides, and a main road on the other. On the side furthest from the road, the main railway line passes. But for those of us who had walked far enough already, there's a way to get round and rest your souls; the UK's oldest miniature railway.

It opened in 1911 and its fortunes have varied over the years, but it's currently enjoying quite a boom. Certainly the busiest place we'd seen in Rhyl. They use real steam engines (most days anyway) so there's always the appeal of getting smoke and soot in your eyes.

For added railway authenticity, we broke down halfway round and had to wait for the engine to cool down.

On the way back to the real Rhyl station, we stopped off for some chips. When I rule the world, I'll pass a law that you must eat chips when you're at the seaside. I didn't feel too guilty about it as the mileage we had done deserved a few calories. We caught the train home, but we'd be back to the North Wales coast.

The next stop along the line after Prestatyn and Rhyl is Abergele. Although it has to share its station with Pensarn. Abergele is unique amongst the North Wales resorts for not having a sandy beach. This probably explains why so few trains stop there. But it doesn't stop the ever-onward march of the holiday caravan; again they were everywhere. This time I was travelling with my children.

Our reasoning for missing out Abergele was two-fold. The next stop had a sandy beach and a zoo. But as the train sped through Abergele, my youngest noticed a sign. "Crazy Golf" it said. Suddenly we were on a two-resort day out.

On arrival at Colwyn Bay station, just outside the doors, a mini-bus painted as a zebra picks you up to take you to the Welsh Mountain Zoo. It lives up to its name in all ways. It's Welsh, on a mountain, and a zoo.

It dropped us by the bear enclosure. We looked in. It was empty. I'm never sure what to do in these circumstances. Should we tell them the bears have escaped? Or do they actually have no bears but hope no one questions it?

We went to see the pandas at Edinburgh Zoo once. When we were outside, they said the pandas had gone in. When we were in, they said the pandas had gone out. I didn't believe they had anything other than a cage of bamboo.

I'm not sure on the exact mileage we walked at the Welsh Mountain Zoo, but I awarded myself bonus mileage for the sheer uphills we did. It appeared to be all uphill. There appeared to be no downhill. Just uphill after uphill.

We saw all the usual zoo animals along with the performing penguins in their own show. We found a picnic bench on a mountainside for our lunch. The views would have been fantastic were it not located in the middle of a bush. Why it was placed there I can't even begin to imagine. Still, it meant no one else was sat there.

After visiting the camels and another look for the bears-still missing-we went to join the queue for the zebra bus back to the station. As luck would have it, the next train called at Abergele & Pensarn, so crazy golf it was.

I'd never been to Abergele before. To be honest I'd not missed much. Aside from the crazy golf, the attached amusement arcade and café, there's really nothing else there. Mind you, the crazy golf was both good and cheap.

Where the sand should be, were rocks and boulders. There was no way you could walk on the beach here. We went back to the station and waited for the next train home.

11 THE ORME IS GREAT

Due to our detour to Abergele, we hadn't actually visited Colwyn Bay. All our Colwyn Bay walking had been uphill at the zoo. We were going to come back, but first, we carried ever onward to Llandudno.

Llandudno's claim to fame is that it has two beaches. The main beach is the most popular, and although it has sandy parts it also has rocky parts. The quieter West Shore Beach is much sandier. It gets two beaches by being on a headland that sticks out into the sea. Although the town part is flat, rising out to sea at one end is The Great Orme. At the other end of the town is a much smaller hill called, with breathtaking originality, The Little Orme.

The Little Orme is the poor relative. Tucked away far from town. No paths up it or round it. No attractions on it. No road on it. In short, no one goes there. There's nothing to go there for.

The Great Orme boasts no fewer than five ways up it. You can, of course, walk. There are a variety of different paths to choose from. You can walk up the road or you can choose from any number of footpaths.

If you've come in your car, you can drive up. If you haven't come in your car, you can still drive up but it involves theft, so isn't encouraged.

You can get the bus up. The service isn't that frequent, but there are several buses a day.

You can get a tram up. These are still the original Victorian trams that run. I don't understand the full physics behind it, but basically the tram going down pulls the other tram up. Due to the distance, you have to get off halfway and board another one. Although these are the original trams and no others have ever run on the line, they are numbered 3,4,5 & 6.

Finally, there is the cable car. The cable car opened in 1969 and the original cars still run now. It doesn't fill you with confidence. However, it can't operate when there are thunderstorms, heavy rain, or the wind speed is above 22mph, which on the Orme is most days. I think they've run about three days in total so far.

Which ever way you get to the top, once there you are rewarded with a panoramic view. Behind you, you can see over Llandudno, in all other directions is the Irish Sea.

Not wanting to miss out on a chance to relieve you of your hard-earned money, there's a café, shop and crazy golf course on the summit. There's also a small children's playground (that's a playground that is small and not a playground for small children) and a small visitor centre.

Partway back down, near the halfway tram station, is a copper mine. This dates back 4,000 years to the Bronze Age. No one knew it was there until they started work to make a car park and literally stumbled into it.

There's an information centre, a short video about it, and then you don your hard hat and head off underground. You "self-guide" your way round the mines, but it's really not hard and you can't get lost. There's a one-way system and it's lit. A feature I guess they didn't have 4,000 years ago.

However, we were here for none of these attractions. We were here to walk. On this trip, my walking companion was my youngest son. The walk we were doing was the road around the Great Orme. This is called Marine Drive.

It's five miles long and is literally just what the doctor ordered. You can drive round it; it's still five miles long, but there's a £3.50 toll for cars. There's also a vintage bus tour that goes round, but as we were there in the height of summer, it had been replaced with an open-top minibus.

It's a one-way road, at least for the first three and a half miles anyway, but the flexibility of walking means you can go either way. But we went the same way as the traffic. They all stopped at the toll booth to pay their way; we just marched on through. It felt good.

The road starts a steady climb. After a bit, we turned round to admire the view behind us. We looked down on the pier jutting out into the sea. It opened in 1878 and is 1234 feet long, which I find strangely pleasing. There is a landing stage at the end where, in years gone by, you could catch a boat to Liverpool or The Isle of Man.

The Pier Pavilion played host to many famous names, including Cliff Richard and Arthur Askey. But a fire in 1994 razed the building to the ground where its remained ever since.

Continuing on our walk, the path continued its slow climb, clinging to the hillside with just the sea to our right. Clinging to the hillside on our left were rock climbers. It seemed a lot of work and effort and they couldn't admire the view as they were facing away from the sea and towards the rocks. But they seemed to be enjoying it.

There were sheep everywhere, clinging to improbably narrow ledges, some halfway up a cliff face as if they were dropped there from above. Some stubbornly sat in the road. I've never understood why lamb is so expensive when there are so many sheep.

The road took a little downhill turn, but it was only so it could rise up further and steeper. There's a turning off to the summit here; drivers can turn off, park at the summit (parking is included in the toll fee) and then come back and carry on if they so wish. Walkers can too, but it's much more effort. On the way to the summit, you pass St Tudno's Church. If you want to see it, but don't fancy the walk, there's a free bus up on Sundays for the service.

Carrying on round Marine Drive, what looks like a castle comes into view. Except it isn't. It's a lighthouse. As it's so high up on the hillside already, they didn't need the usual tall tower. It first shone on 1st December 1862 and every single night thereafter till March 22nd 1985 when they gave up. It's now a holiday B&B.

The last climb on the walk is after the lighthouse. You can see the building you're aiming for, sitting on the hilltop. This, you assume, must be the end. A very pleasant walk. The end is in sight. It's only when you arrive and see the sign "Halfway House. Rest & Be Thankful Café," that the disappointment sets in.

We rested and were thankful. Then trudged on. The problem with this walk of course, is that you can't abandon it part way.

The good news though is that it's downhill all the way now. Once you've rounded the headland, giving you views to Puffin Island and across to Conwy, you can see, down at sea level, the remains of The Royal Artillery Coastal Gunnery School, opening here in 1940. At its peak, over 700 personnel were stationed here. There's nothing but a few lumps of concrete now. Nature is slowly taking over.

There's another castle-looking building down below. This used to be, till it closed, The Railway Convalescent Home. Railway workers could stay here whilst convalescing. People don't do convalescing anymore, so it shut. This sort of place would have suited me when I came out of hospital, but you're just expected to fend for yourself these days.

The road below now becomes "Millionaires Row" with big posh houses and their big posh gardens running to the sea. It was said

Cliff Richard used to own one of these. It was the one with a tennis court in the garden. Either he no longer owns it, or he's fallen on hard times. The tennis court is overgrown and the house looks like it's seen better days.

There still appear to be plenty of millionaires though. With new big posh houses being built with new big posh gardens, running down to the sea. You miss these views if you drive round in the car. We stop to peer over the wall a little more closely and take it all in. It is a lot windier on this side. But the views are still impressive.

We carry on to the end and the road comes out by Llandudno West Shore Beach. It's a hot sunny day and the beach is full of families making the most of it. There's an ice cream van parked up, he doesn't take cards, I don't have cash. He gives me directions to a cash point. On the way back, we see a road train about to depart to the town centre. We hop on and splash the cash on that instead.

When I visited Llandudno with Cath, we took an open-top bus tour which took in both beaches, along with Deganway and Conway. We alighted at West Shore Beach for an ice cream and the last bus of the day came near to the bus stop, but went right round a roundabout and headed back, leaving us stranded. I've never had much luck with ice cream here.

After alighting the road train (you only ever alight trains, no one alights a car), we strolled wearily down the main sea front. The Mostyn family have held sway in Llandudno for as long as anyone can remember. To this day, all the buildings on the sea front can only be painted pastel colours, from a limited palette, all approved by the Mostyns. The family also decreed that no building can be higher than the width of the road it is on. Rather than having very short buildings, this does give Llandudno some very wide roads.

We had an ice cream on the sea front, soaked up a bit of sun and wearily headed off to Llandudno railway station for the train home.

12 RETURN TO WALES

Colwyn Bay continued to elude us. It was time to put this right. We got off the train at Colwyn Bay; Cath, my youngest and me. We headed down to the sea. We were stopped at some barriers by a security guard. The sea front was out of bounds as there was a car rally taking place. This was unexpected.

Instead, we walked parallel to the sea, but unable to see or hear it. We could have been anywhere. Or at least anywhere with a street full of rally cars.

We walked onwards and came to a road to the beach that was open; finally, we'd arrived. Admittedly we were now more in Rhos than Colwyn Bay, but let us not get bogged down in technicalities.

The people of Rhos had cashed in on the rally being in town. There were people dressed as cars and a couple of stalls. There was also a model racetrack, with remote control cars being 'driven' by hapless but enthusiastic members of the public with steering wheels behind.

We stayed to watch, and were about to move on when the commentator said, "Take your places ready for the next race. It's free." At the mention of free we went straight round to have a go.

It really is very difficult to control a car by steering it whilst looking down at it on a track. Each twist and turn changes the way you need to turn the wheel. We were hapless and hopeless. But we made up for it in our enthusiasm. Needless to say, none of the three of us won.

Rhos is a small pleasant town, but it doesn't have many seaside attractions. But we did find a crazy golf course. It was into September now, and it looked for all the world like it was shut. The kiosk where you'd clearly pay and buy ice creams was closed and the chairs were stacked upside down on the tables. Always a sure sign it wasn't going to open anytime soon. But then we noticed a bit of paper in the window. "If closed, pay in the pub." This seemed an unusual approach, but we went into the pub, and sure enough they had a rack of clubs and a basket of balls.

We had a very enjoyable game. It was just us. Unusually there were two holes on one…hole. You all tee off at the same place but then the course goes both left and right so you can choose to putt into either. This did make the hole more fun.

We continued on our walk round Rhos. It was a small pleasant town, which appeared to have almost forgotten it was on the coast, despite a lovely sandy beach.

We stopped at the solitary beachside kiosk for some chips. They were lovely and the kiosk was very busy as a result.

As part of the car rally, there was a small air show taking place over the sea. We watched the planes flying in loops and in carefully rehearsed manoeuvres which appeared to show the planes passing improbably close to each other at great speed.

We strolled back down the seafront to Colwyn Bay. I remembered coming here as a child. Although I can't have been that old, I remember there being a few children's rides and a pier. Then in the 1980s they ripped the heart out of Colwyn Bay and replaced it with its own bypass. The A55.

They say you can't stop progress. But progress stopped Colwyn Bay. Instead of people driving the coast road and stopping off at Colwyn Bay, they now drive the A55 and don't even notice Colwyn Bay is there at all. It separates town from sea. It's hard to think of a single redeeming feature of it for the people of Colwyn Bay.

As tourists stopped coming, so the pier fell into disrepair. In its heyday, the pier hosted performances by such names as Motorhead, Slade and Madness.

In 1987, only a few years after the A55 was completed, the pier was suffering so badly the seaward extremity was closed off to the public. In 1991, there was a fire in the pier buildings, from which only the insurance document survived. Now, you wouldn't know there had ever been a pier here.

Wandering around seaside towns was providing fresh air and exercise. But it was time to get some proper mileage in now.

13 THE HERITAGE TRAIL

Cath lives near Cannock Chase and we often go over for a walk around. Various different coloured signposts take you on varying lengths of walk. For the more adventurous there are mountain bike trails too. We always ended up at the visitor centre and tea rooms after our rambles.

It was over a coffee and cake, after a particularly exhilarating walk across the Chase, that Cath spotted a leaflet for the Heritage Trail. A walk, it claimed, from Rugeley to Cannock, passing through Cannock Chase. There was a vague map on the leaflet and everything about it suggested this was a proper, well-marked route. We both wanted to do it. So we did.

The plan was cunningly simply. Train to Cannock, walk the 10 mile "heritage trail" back to Rugeley and train back home.

First problem. Due to overnight flooding, there were no trains to Cannock. Instead a minibus turned up, with a driver who oozed no confidence at all that he knew what he was doing. We told him we wanted Cannock. He said he called at all stations. Strangely, all the other passengers stayed at the station and it was just us as we set off.

He promptly turned into an industrial estate that was clearly a dead end. Having decided that station was too hard to find, we set off for the next. The SatNav had different ideas about where Hednesford Station was compared to the road signs. The driver took a combination of the two, and ignored my helpful suggestion of, "Look! There it is," as we did two laps of the town. Eventually, we parked under a "Hednesford Station" sign and the driver waited for us to move. When we didn't, he said, "Isn't this Cannock Station?"

Reprogramming SatNav, we set off again. We were following road signs for Cannock Station and were within sight of it, when he realised that wasn't what SatNav was saying. We did a u-turn, drove onto a housing estate and he dropped us there.

At that point, we thought that was the worst thing that could go wrong. How wrong we were! Having, eventually, made it to Cannock Station, all the trail literature promised a well-signed route of level paths suitable for wheelchairs and pushchairs. There was a map at the station entrance, but it didn't actually tell you where the trail was. A trip down the road found a trail sign (on a three-way junction) at a drunken angle, that could have been pointing in any direction.

We found a country park, thought that could be it, but the information board made no mention of the trail. However, a couple, who looked local, were just arriving. We asked them. We told them we were walking to Rugeley on the Heritage Trail and we were after some directions. They eyed us with some suspicion and had never heard of the trail. Although the man offered the comforting words, "Rugeley is a long way. A VERY long way."

However, we spotted a Heritage Trail post, although not offering any directions. But, as the path was straight, we couldn't go wrong-could we? We followed the path till we found two ladies walking dogs. We asked them about the trail. I could say many things about the ladies, but as I'm nice, let's just say I think they were confused. They said to, "Carry on, go up the steps and at the top turn right. Or left." It was the last part that, if I'm honest, did worry me a bit.

There were no signposts or maps to go any other way, so up the steps we went. At the top was a main road, where the path clearly went straight ahead across the road, and down some more steps. Reflecting back on it now, I should have raised a concern that this clearly wasn't pushchair and wheelchair friendly. But I just thought the families and disabled of Cannock were more adventurous. We carried on regardless.

At each fork in the path, there continued to be no signage at all. We did ask other people walking. None had heard of the trail and all looked suitably impressed we were walking to Rugeley. Eventually, we emerged onto a road, and found ourselves nearly at Hednesford. Surely we could pick up the trail again here?

Although we arrived in Hednesford from an unconventional direction, we found a Heritage Trail sign in the High Street. And what a lovely High Street it is, if you want to place a bet or order a takeaway. We carried onto the station and to our surprise and delight found not only a map, but our first signpost too. Unfortunately, the sign to Rugeley pointed to a T junction with no further clue where to go. We did a couple more laps of Hednesford, but on foot this time, waving to the minibus driver who was going round again on his way back.

Eventually, we worked out the path went through Tesco and Hednesford Park. We stopped in Tesco for the toilet. Being hot and grumpy at this point, I put the backpack, with lunch in, on the sinks whilst I washed and dried my hands. Oblivious to the fact that the backpack had triggered the automatic taps and our lunch was slowly getting wet. We ploughed on through the park.

Although there were no signposts of course, there was a leaflet about it pinned to a board, which did promise the route went through the park and had had a lottery grant to fund signposts. I smell a scam. We came out of the park and onto a road, and with no clue at all, turned left. Then, against all the odds, there were some signposts all the way to Cannock Chase Visitor Centre!

We stopped there for a soggy sandwich, and found the Great War Hut open. I'd have called it The Perfectly OK War Hut to be honest. But it was laid out as it would have been in The Great War, and there were very enthusiastic volunteers to tell you all you ever wanted to know, and much, much more too.

Buoyed on by the recent signpost frenzy, we set off again. After the success of getting to Cannock Chase with signposts, we were getting overconfident with signs. However, the trail committee soon rectified this by providing no more signs. We, of course, soon arrived at a T junction with no signpost. We knew the next major point on the route to be Birches Valley Visitor Centre. It felt like it was right, so we went right. We met a couple coming from that direction. We asked what was that way and if the visitor centre was that way. They said they didn't know what was that way, and they were looking for the visitor centre too. We turned round, but the path seemed to loop back from where we had come from. So we turned back again. We met another couple and asked them. They told us the same thing. No one knew where that path went, but we all knew it didn't go to the Visitor Centre. We turned round again and came to a turning, where someone had put a sign to the Visitor Centre. They've probably been sacked now for gross misconduct.

Suddenly we came to a five-way fork. There was even a signpost! One way promised Cannock was 6 miles away (although, interestingly, not the way we had come from) whilst Rugeley was a mere 4 miles in one of the other directions. However, the angle of the sign made it very unclear which one of the four other ways it was. Having got used to making pot-luck choices all day, we did so again, and got lucky again.

Finally, we turned a corner and saw the welcome sight of Rugeley Power Station. A sign promised Rugeley was now just 2 miles away. We ploughed on. Obviously, there was another fork in the path without a signpost. This time we made the wrong choice, ended up not seeing another sign, and had to use google maps to get back to the station.

Neither the start nor end of the walk was marked in any way. But we did get a train. If anyone says, "Let's do the Heritage Trail?" to you, please just say no. Or invest in an ordnance survey map.

What we needed was a well signposted walk. The hunt was on.

14 THE WIRRAL WAY

The Wirral way runs for twelve miles between two railway stations. It was originally a railway line, but as it didn't particularly go anywhere much, it was closed. More people walk and cycle it now than ever caught a train on it.

The beauty of walking an old railway line is that it's flat, and very easy to follow. It starts (or ends if you're heading the other way) at Hooton railway station. Hooton Station has four platforms. Two are used by the regular services to and from Liverpool and onwards to Ellesmere Port and Chester. Another sees occasional use for services which start or end at Hooton, and the fourth is used so rarely, it isn't even numbered.

Mind you, it had been used just a few days before our visit. By someone who doesn't worry about platform numbers as she has her own train. Yes, the Royal Train had deposited Her Majesty at Hooton Station just a few days before. Goodness knows what she did there. As far as I could see there was nothing for miles. Maybe she hired a bike.

Although the unnumbered platform is a dead end, the track continues through the platform for quite some way. It was down here they pulled the Royal Train that night for Her Majesty to sleep on.

The unnumbered platform is the one you have to use to get on and off the station. Quite why the station is arranged that way is a mystery, but we made our way across all four platforms and out onto the road. We then used the road bridge to cross back over all four platforms and onto the start of the Wirral Way.

There is bike hire available at Hooton and they, of course, promote the Wirral Way to ride them on. The Heritage Trail really could learn some lessons here. You can hire bikes one-way and leave them at West Kirby at the other end.

I was with Cath again for this walk, and as neither of us had ridden a bike for over thirty years, we decided we'd stick with walking. Ironically, the last train to carry a passenger over the line was the Royal Train in 1957. Maybe she was just visiting for old times sake.

The path is, of course, at ground level so initially you have the wall of the platform on your left, but once clear of the station it opens out to countryside on all sides.

Several people passed us on bikes. Many on their own, but some on the hire bikes. At this point the path is quite narrow and they would ring their bells as a signal to move out of the way, as apparently, it's impossible for a cyclist to stop and give way. Sometimes we wouldn't hear the bell, being lost in conversation with each other. The cyclists could then get quite shirty and shout "move" or other things. Generally, and I know it's wrong to make sweeping generalisations, the more lycra a cyclist wore, the more hurry they were in and the ruder they were. Those in jeans on the hire bikes were generally more considerate. Indeed, we even wondered if they didn't enjoy the break when they had to stop to pass us, often engaging in conversation with us and adopting a carefree approach to getting any exercise.

Not too far into the walk, you come to the former station of Hadlow Road. Here it is always 1956. The station has been restored to its former glory. There's a waiting room, toilets, ticket office, signal box, luggage and milk churns on the platform. Indeed everything there was in 1956, except for trains. There are more people now too.

We stopped for a nosey around. They really have made it very nice. It's a lot nicer than many stations that do have trains. If it wasn't for the fact we'd just walked where the track should be, I'd have happily waited for a train. But we still had a long way to go.

We carried on. The path widened out, and horse riders got their own section. Although we didn't see any. The cyclists and pedestrians still had to share though. Railway lines are often straight and the walk stretched off into the distance.

Eventually we came to the town of Parkgate. We diverted off the path and down to the front. Parkgate is, in many ways, a seaside town. It has a front; it has ice cream shops. The thing it lacks, is sea. If you walk down the front, where the sea should be is salt marsh. It's never been sea, but it did used to be a port on the River Dee. The Dee gradually silted up and Parkgate got the raw deal. On the spring high tide, water still flows over the marsh and Parkgate gets to enjoy being a seaside town, just for the day.

It's quite a sight and lots of people turn out for it apparently. But we weren't there in the right season so we just had to take their word for it.

One thing Parkgate continues to offer is locally made ice cream. There are now three shops all selling their own ice cream. And all claiming to be the original. They offer a wide range of flavours, some traditional, and others less so. I went for tangerine flavour and it was very nice.

We ate them out on the front. A man came over to us and struck up conversation. We were clearly tourists and he felt the need to let us know that he was a local. He told us that what we could see on the other side of the Dee was in fact Wales, and in particular Shotton. In other words, when we were on the train to Wales, we would see Parkgate. On cue, a train trundled through Shotton on the far bank.

He then had to go to get his bus home. But I felt it had brightened his day to impart this knowledge on us. We took a last look at Shotton, finished our ice creams and headed back to the path.

The path continued ever onwards. A straight path heading off into the distance as far as the eye could see. Still, at least there was a path and it was clearly marked. Over to our left, every so often, we caught a glimpse of the river and eventually the sea.

At Thurstaston there is a visitor centre. It's located on the original station platform but is a new building. There were open spaces, and families sat on benches and the grass, eating picnics. There was a twelve-mile path next to them but most had wandered no more than twelve yards from the car park. I suspect many didn't even know the path was there.

We stopped to use the toilets. Whilst I was waiting for Cath, I studied the animal and plant information board. I always look at these and think I should make more effort to appreciate what I'm walking through. But as soon as I set off, I promptly forget and just end up thinking, "That's a nice yellow flower."

There was a café but it had those wipe down plastic tablecloths which never improve a place. We bought a drink to take outside. We sat out and enjoyed the sunshine whilst resting our weary feet.

Realising we couldn't get home from here without walking, we set back off. Maybe because we'd had a rest, we'd lost enthusiasm now. The walk became tedious. Just a path stretching off to the horizon. We ploughed on.

For the final stretch into West Kirby, houses back onto the track which adds a bit of interest. They have views to the sea from upstairs and many have balconies to take advantage of this.

Eventually, we arrived at West Kirby and headed to the beach. Being a hot, sunny, Sunday afternoon, the beach was heaving with families. Yet strangely it had less in the way of attractions than Parkgate had. But the obvious bonus of sea and sand.

We got a drink from the sole seaside kiosk and collapsed onto the beach exhausted. Having enjoyed the delights of West Kirby, we walked back to the station, passing the bike hire return, and got the train home.

15 RETURN TO DEVON

I've always fancied myself as a Royal Marine. Clearly I have the looks and fitness: almost. There is a commando training camp on the banks of the River Exe and when I passed on the train, they were covered head to toe in mud and climbing out of the river mud bed back to camp. My plan was a bit less energetic and a lot less messy.

I was travelling back to Exmouth. This time I was going to follow the Exe Estuary Trail, which follows the Exe all the way to Exeter, before crossing over and following the opposite bank of the Exe all the way to Dawlish.

My plan was simplicity itself. As the train line also follows the Exe, I'd get off at Exmouth and walk back as far as I felt like before getting a train back.

The full walk is sixteen and a half miles, so if planning to do the full walk it's best to bring sandwiches. I hadn't got any food, but then I seriously doubted I'd walk the full trail. Not when it passes so many railway stations.

I'd made an early start and alighted at Exmouth just before 8am. I left the station through the car park and found the path next to the railway line which it follows all the way to Lympstone. Lympstone is a pretty village, which was just waking up when I got there. The railway passes over on a bridge and a train went over it as I went under it.

Having just missed a train, and not having done that much walking, I decided I'd carry on rather than get a train back from here. But the path passes the station so I stopped for a look anyway. There's not much to it. A couple of seats and a bus shelter. I pressed on.

The path up to this point had previously existed. It had been upgraded and a lot of work had been done to it, but from Lympstone Village station it was a new path. Laid out to give pedestrians and cyclists enough room each without the need for bike bells going off all the time.

The path is very popular with both cyclists and pedestrians. Its easy access to villages and public transport clearly a big draw. A safe, traffic-free environment proving a big hit.

The marine training camp has its own station, Lympstone Commando. Before the path was constructed, the only access from the platforms was direct into the camp. There are railway signs on a red background, conveying the serious message that only those with business at the camp could use the station. Although the message ended there, you got the feeling they had wanted to add, "Anyone with no business at the camp will be shot on sight." There was a sentry guard hut on the platform although it was unmanned when I passed.

Since the Exe Estuary Trail has been built between the station and the training camp, it now seems unnecessary to ban everyone else as there is access onto the path. Indeed, the marines have to cross the path to get between the camp and the station. It is not often you can use the word 'camp' and 'marine' in the same sentence.

There was a train due and I wondered if I could pass myself off as a marine and get on it. But I bottled out. I knew I'd be caught and interrogated; going for a walk because the doctor said so just didn't sound like a good enough excuse and I would crack under the pressure.

I did wait for the train to leave, then, when no one was looking, sneaked onto the platform. Just quickly. Before guiltily leaving. With the right upbringing, it's amazing what you can feel guilty about.

The path follows the camp boundary. There's an assault course and the recruits were being put through their paces by someone shouting at them. It occurred to me that maybe the high fence with barbed wire on the top wasn't to keep the likes of me out, but to keep them in. If I was them I'd be trying to escape.

The path continues to Exton station. This is a request stop, so you have to put your arm out, as you would a bus, to stop it. Despite this, not all the trains will stop anyway. Some will pass through regardless. The next one I could stop was nearly an hour away. I pressed on.

At Exton was The Puffing Billy pub. It looked very nice and I would have stopped for food had it been open, but it wasn't; it still being too early, despite it being 11 o'clock.

The path, due to houses and a general lack of space, does follow the road here for a short way. But it's a quiet road and no cars passed me. Soon enough the dedicated path returns and you're crossing the River Clyst. You can take a small diversion to Darts Farm. At one time purely a farm, now keen to release tourists of their holiday spending money. They sell farm products, upmarket household items, even camping gear, but it's their butchers and meat department that they are best known for.

The path continues to Topsham and handily passes the station. As there was a train due, I decided to call it a day and head back. Although the line from Exeter to Exmouth is largely single track, to permit the half hourly frequency, two trains have to pass each other and Topsham is the place they do it.

It also means all the trains have to stop, no need to stick your arm out. In the olden days, drivers would get a token to use the single line. It was a fail-safe system. If you had the token, you couldn't meet another train as there was only one token. Unless of course the other driver had made a mistake. These days it's done electronically. It might be safer, but some of the romance is gone. No longer does the signalman (and it was always a man) lean out of the window of the signal box, offering the token to the driver, who would lean out of his window with blatant disregard for health and safety and grab it.

Now they simply press a button and the computer knows what train is where. That's progress for you. Mind you, I didn't mind, I was just grateful for the sit down.

A few days later and I walk from Dawlish Warren to Starcross again. Then I carry on down the Exe Estuary Trail rather than getting the ferry. It goes off road now and slots in on the edge of Powderham Castle, the home of the Earl of Devon. It's well worth a visit in its own right, but I didn't have time today. I was heading to the pub.

The Turf Locks pub cannot, so they claim, be accessed by car. Only by foot or boat. I'd come by canoe before (no, really) so now it was time to come by foot. The first thing that surprises many a first-time visitor, who has either had to walk or paddle to get to this no cars pub, is how many cars there are. Indeed, there was a lorry there making a delivery when I walked up.

What they mean when they say you can't get there by car, is just that. They don't mean cars can't get there, just you can't get there by car. There's just a private road to it and no real parking. The private road is hard to find even when you know where it is.

It's a very nice pub and does very nice food. I sat outside and enjoyed some whilst I waited for the ferry. It runs every half hour. Near enough. It takes fifteen minutes to cross to Topsham.

On arrival at Topsham, I picked up the trail again heading towards Exeter. It emerged onto the road at Countess Wear which is still a swing bridge to let tall ships pass, although no one I spoke to can ever remember it opening to ships. That might be because when they built the M5, they didn't build it tall enough to allow ships under, so there's no real point in them passing under Countess Wear.

I could have continued into Exeter City Centre. I could have crossed over and walked back to the Turf Locks. Or I could, and did, walk to the bus stop and get the bus back. Satisfied, I'd done most of the trail.

16 THE WINTER

Walking is all well and good in nice weather, but the shine quickly rubs off in the wet and cold. Consequently, it's harder to get exercise in the winter. Wrapping up in layers is all well and good, but it's miserable when you have your hood up and can only hear the scratch of the material against your ear.

When Becky asked me if I wanted to do Couch to 5K with her, I thought it would be good. I'd never really run before so this sounded the ideal way to start. Running would also keep me warm.

The only problem was that we'd missed week one. But the running club who organised it assured us it wouldn't be a problem. We turned up at the club, eager to go on Wednesday night. What I hadn't anticipated was to have two homework runs each week to do on my own.

This week's run at the club was run a minute then walk a minute, ten times. They had a track which made it better. When everyone is running in a loop, you can never be at the back, there are always people behind you. Even if they're actually the people in front of you.

Gareth was the run leader. He was a happy chappy who loved running and his infectious enthusiasm rubbed off on us. There were around 150 people all on the journey from couch to 5K. He started us off with a warm-up. To me, this was cheating.

We were going to run for ten minutes (albeit interspersed with ten minutes of walking) but the warm-up added another two minutes of running. This was unfair.

Warm-up complete, we started our first minutes run. It's amazing how long a minute can be. Eventually, after what felt like ten minutes, Gareth shouted, "You're halfway. Just 30 more seconds." REALLY?? Becky was enjoying herself and hadn't broken a sweat. I was close to collapse.

The whistle blew and we all stopped running to walk for a minute. This minute was much faster. In no time at all, Gareth blew the whistle to start running again. Off we went.

When I'd had my bypass, they had deflated my lungs. In intensive care, they kept making me breathe fully in and fully out to fully inflate them again. Right now it felt like it hadn't worked.

By the fifth minute, people were looking at me as they went past me. I must have been a sight to behold. Sweat dripping off me from every pore. My face the colour of a tomato, but slightly more red and my lungs on the verge of collapse. Still, my heart was doing just fine.

I battled on and did all the ten minutes. Just. When I got back to Becky's, I was unable to speak for quite some time and just sat there recovering. Gradually, my face returned to a normal colour, my lungs were full and I regained the power of speech.

The homework was to do that again twice more before the next week's club run. I did, under cover of darkness, and each time it got easier. Mind you, I didn't do the extra warm-up running. But I did the cool down stretches.

The next week, we were up to ninety seconds of running with sixty seconds walking. Each week, the running time went up and the walking time went down. But I got better at it. I stopped going red. I went longer before my lungs collapsed. I was able to walk and talk back at Becky's afterwards.

My youngest son started running my homework runs with me. He also started coming to the track on the club nights. We'd leave our water bottles near the club house, and if we wanted a drink he'd run off round the track, get the bottle, carry on round the track and give it to us. Before running off again to put it back. He could do three laps of the track to my one. What it is to be young.

Eventually it was time to run 5K. Gareth had made us register for the local Parkrun which used the park and old railway line next to the club. The course is simple; run 2.5K turn round and run back. This was a new Parkrun and didn't officially start till the following week. We were the guinea pigs to try it out.

We were told there was a steward and a cone at the 2.5K mark. Run round them and come back. We were told to look out for low hanging branches and speed humps. After the briefing was over, Gareth asked what we had to look out for.
"Steward and a cone." I replied. Apparently, the answer was low hanging branches and speed humps.

I didn't come last. But I did finish some way behind Becky, who in turn finished some way behind my youngest son. Cath sacrificed a better time for herself to run with me. But I did finish.

I usually had to work on Saturdays so doing a normal Parkrun wasn't an option. But one week I was off, so volunteered to steward.

It was 08:30 on a Saturday morning. Normal people are still in bed. Normally I'm at work, but for one week only I was in a field with 150 odd people, and I was the only one not in Lycra. It was the 19th Wammy Parkrun. Strangely, I was last there 20 weeks ago. Prior to the coach to 5K, I'd never so much as run for a bus before.

At each point along the way, where there's a path on and off the route, a steward is stationed to ensure no runners escape. One of these was my location. I'd never stewarded before, and armed with my hi-viz jacket and a "Keep Left" sign, I headed off.

Your steward lanyard gives your postcode location, the postcode location of all the other stewards, a list of phone numbers and details of what to do in an emergency. Which is quite good, as my natural reaction would be to panic.

I was around a third of the way (and therefore also two thirds of the way) along the course. It wasn't long before the fastest were with me. They mainly wore 10k, half-marathon and marathon tops from their previous event runs. It's a bit like wearing a Reading festival top to Glastonbury. It lets any lightweights in the crowd know you do this all the time.

I clapped as the first came past, but a sole clapper didn't sound right; clapping is a community thing. So I offered verbal encouragement instead, and helpful things like "see you on the other side" before realising the unfortunate double meaning and switching to "see you on the way back."

A lady then appeared onto the path with her dog. A big, hairy beast intent on sniffing at me. The dog not the lady. She deftly crossed in front of the runners, and onto the far side of the path. The main crowd of runners then followed, coming along thick and fast, but mainly fast.

There were runners of all shapes and sizes, parents with children, parents trying to keep up with children, those who looked like they could easily do it again, those for whom every step was clearly an effort. But all fairly serious. No fancy dress. No one with a washing machine strapped onto their back.

Then the tail-walking steward passed. Their job is to ensure no one gets left behind; as long as they don't step over a collapsed body all is good. Only enough time to turn my 'Keep Left' sign to point the other way, and the leader comes thundering back through. Completed in 17.26mins, it's a new personal best for them.

But disaster struck. The lady and the big, hairy beast were now on opposite sides of the path to each other, and a retractable lead stretched across the path in between them, in the runners' way. I thought about shouting "mind the lead" but worried the runner would misinterpret this to mean someone was catching him up so to run faster. I didn't want to be the steward on duty the time someone fell headfirst over a dog lead. Thankfully, the lady realised in time and hit the button to retract the lead, but as the dog was so big, nothing happened. However, the lead did its job, dragging the lady across the path and disaster was averted.

Call me simple if you want, but I hadn't expected thanks from the runners! I was amazed how they said, "Thank you steward," as they passed, and it's appreciated. I guess without the stewards, they can't run. Mind you, I'd look pretty stupid stewarding without the runners, so it cuts both ways.

The return runners were more spread out, and you could tell the latest Couch to 5K graduates, as they swung their arms back and forth-not across-with their thumbs pointing up, as coached by Gareth. He'd be very proud.

You may think that the finish line is the end, but oh no. As 5K isn't quite far enough, most people carry on (admittedly walking) to the Newcastle Athletics Club clubhouse for 'Ken's Café' and a chat. The really keen do a few laps of the track too.

17 CACHE IN THE ATTIC

Geocaching came about when someone realised that GPS locations, that were previously solely for use by governments and the military, were available to the public.

Quite how the leap of thought then came about that this meant you could hide Tupperware, isn't recorded. But come about it did.

In the early days, you needed special GPS devices. Nowadays, any smartphone and the geocaching app will do. In simple terms, anyone can hide anything anywhere. There are, of course, a few rules, but essentially that's it. The minimum requirement is that whatever you hide must contain a piece of paper to sign; the log. A signature on the log is the only official way to say you've found a geocache. But obviously, to keep a track, you log it on the website too.

Unfound caches on the map are green. Log one as found and it turns into a yellow smiley face for you. Log one that you did not find (DNF) and it shows you a blue sad face. There's something strangely satisfying about seeing the map fill with yellow smiley faces.

We started off getting some easy ones. Large containers not hidden too difficultly. Some people go to a lot of trouble to hide their containers. You get them disguised as logs or stones, even leaves or snails. As our experience increased, so did our caching adventures.

The biggest adventure we went on involved walking the canal all the way from Macclesfield in Cheshire to Kidsgrove in Staffordshire. 121 caches in total. And a very long walk.

We'd planned the day meticulously. We didn't want anything going wrong. We had a phone each, we had a spare charger each. We had a GPS device each. We'd written each cache, and its hint to find it, down in a notebook. We wanted a full house.

We caught the first train of the day to Macclesfield as the first cache in the trail is by the station. The first few then lead you down to the canal. They are all easy finds. On a trail with lots to find, people don't want to be spending ages finding them and not get them all.

The caches are generally the same; a 35mm film canister, often placed in a purpose built wire holder, just out of sight in a hedge or a tree or behind a wall.

We marked them off as we went, find, after find. Then we found a slightly harder one. The wire holder was attached to the underside of a bridge over the canal. It was too high to reach from the ground, the bridge too deep to be able to reach it from the bridge. In the end, we were able to push it out of the holder using a stick.

The problem now was to get it back. We made a few failed attempts. Really we knew they were never going to work. In the end we attached the cache to the stick with a hair bobble, slid it in the holder then slid the bobble off on the side of the holder. Perfect.

We carried on. Find after find. No missing ones, none that eluded us. We left the canal at Congleton railway station. It is next to the canal and although not actually part of the trail, it seemed silly to not find an extra cache whilst so close.

We trotted over the bridge; steps were a novelty after the endless miles of canal towpath. With a lot of metal and the overhead electric cables, the GPS reading was all over the place. We eventually narrowed it down to a corner between the platform and the car park.

I rummaged around in the undergrowth. My caching buddy for the day suddenly shouted, "Found it!"
I stood up and cracked my head on the corner of a metal sign. "Ouch!" I exclaimed.
"You ok?"
I could feel blood trickling down my forehead. My buddy appeared by my side, cache in hand.
"I'm hurt," I said.
"Oh. Sign the log and I'll put it back." It obviously didn't look as bad as it felt, but I was too weak to argue.
"It still hurts," I said on their return.
"Wuss."
We went back to the canal and carried on the trail. I barely mentioned my life-threatening injury again for the rest of the day. Maybe just once or twice.

We got to Kidsgrove without further incident and with a full complement of found caches. The canal handily has an exit up to the station car park. We wandered exhausted onto Kidsgrove station.

We went on all sorts of caching walks. The good thing about geocaching is that the children will come for a walk as they don't realise they're walking. They are just after the next cache.

One Sunday afternoon, my two boys and I were on a trail in the Staffordshire countryside. We had parked the car and were doing a circular walk. We only had one more to get. The public footpath took us through a field.

We walked through the field and into the next one. The cache was just in the field beyond. A bit of woodland and back to the car. As we entered the field before the cache, intending to follow the path diagonally across the field to the gate we could see was open, we went down a small dip. Then we could see it staring at us. A bull.

There was no mistaking it. It was definitely a bull and not a cow. But just to be sure, I looked for udders. There were none. Not wanting to instil a sense of panic in the children, but not wanting to stay in a field with a bull either, I just gently said, "Should we go the other way?"
"Yes!" They both said very quickly.
We turned and walked gently back out of the field so as not to alarm the bull.

I did quickly look back just to see if it was following us. It had its head down. Not in an about to graze sort of way, but in an about to charge sort of way.

I couldn't think how a bull might kill you, but I didn't want to find out either.
"Are you allowed to put bulls in a field with a public footpath?" asked my youngest.
Good question. I'm sure there must be laws about it. You can't have people being killed by animals whilst on a right of way, surely. Mind you, not all farmers are friendly to walkers.

We made it to the gate but the gate was tied open. The bull had full access to the next field. This seemed very reckless. Particularly as we were now in the next field. We moved down the field hidden by the hedge. Where previously we had meticulously kept to the public footpaths, we now no longer cared and just wanted to be safe. Who ties gates open?

I could definitely sense movement the other side of the hedge. My heart was pounding, my head was sweating, my bowels were keen to get involved. "This is fun," I said. It was meant to keep the children calm, but I was also trying to keep myself calm.

At the other end of the field was another gate secured open. We tentatively went through. To the right, the path led down to the road and freedom. To the left the cache. And bull.

Although no one had said anything, there was a tacit understanding that we weren't going to get the cache. The problem now, was the bull had clearly been tracking us and had come to meet us.

We retreated through the uncloseable gate. There was no other immediately obvious way out of the field we were now in. But then our saviour rode into view.

The farmer was on a quad bike. I assumed he was patrolling his fields, or whatever it is farmers do. I was about to explain why we were in this field and not on the path, when he shouted across at us,
"The bull has escaped!"
We already knew, but at least it explained why the bull was on the path.
"Stay here," the farmer carried on, "I'll see if I can get him back into the right field."
I thought about suggesting that keeping the gates shut may help, but thought better of it.
"Hide behind the hedge."
He really wasn't filling me with confidence.

We waited nervously, half crouching, behind a hedge. The bull didn't strike me as easily fooled by a hedge, but I was willing to give it a go.

The farmer came back with fear in his eyes.
"The bull is very angry."
It was nice to know I'd correctly identified it both as a bull and as being angry.
"For your own safety, get out now. Follow the path to the bottom of the field and climb over the fence onto the road."
Now didn't seem the time to ask what an angry bull might do to

us.

I wanted to appear calm in front of the children, as if an angry bull chasing you really isn't anything to worry about. But I couldn't help myself. My amble had become a trot, with a little panicked skip step thrown in, presumably in the hope of confusing the bull.

If Usain Bolt had been with us, we'd have beaten him to the fence. Maybe Olympian training should include being chased by an angry bull. We scaled the fence and landed on the safety of the road. Quite why a flimsy wooden fence afforded us comfort, I don't know. I couldn't see it being much of an obstacle to an angry bull.

We turned round to confirm with the farmer we were now safe. We saw the sign on the fence then. 'Bull loose in field. Do not enter.' No wonder it had escaped, all the gates were tied open.

Undeterred, after our bull experience we decided to hide our own caches. We looked round the house for suitable containers. We found some Tupperware and a few old film canisters in the loft. Then bought more off Amazon.

We laid a trail on a disused railway line behind our house, now converted to a walkway. A nice level walk and no bulls. Perfect. There is usually a race to be the first to find a new geocache and there was a flurry of activity when they first went live on the website. Soon things settled down to a few finds each weekend if the weather was nice. Some people doing odd ones. Some doing the whole trail.

We did other trails, but carefully planned our routes to avoid any fields. Particularly any fields that might contain bulls. We were soon able to wrack up an impressive number of finds. And plenty of exercise too, the main point of course.

18 RUN FOR THE HILLS

I'd kept up the running during the summer too. With a family membership to the club, both Cath and my youngest son came too. The other children were less enthusiastic.

They held separate times for the children, and the club didn't do family running altogether, so we used to go for our own runs.

After the Couch to 5K course, Gareth ran an improvers session, taking over the same time slot. This suited us as we were all new to running. Then over the summer, Gareth went on holiday. We had to join the regular groups.

This was much more intense. Some of these people were serious runners; they competed at county level. We'd all set off together round the track, but when I was halfway round they'd be thundering past me on their second lap.

Track etiquette was that you'd keep to the inside and move to the outside if you wanted to run past someone. I only ever saw the inside of the track. They were always polite and would shout encouragement as they passed.

Not only were they faster and fitter but they had breath left for conversation too. Mind you, they were younger and hadn't had heart surgery. That was my excuse and I was sticking to it.

Eventually, the summer passed and Gareth returned, along with the improvers session. One session, we left the comfort of the track for the adjacent walkway that used to be a railway line.

Where the parkrun is held. It was a 16:14 session.

In a 16:14 session, the idea is that you run for 16 minutes, then turn round and run back in 14. If you've paced yourself correctly, you'll be back where you started. It's all about pace. No good exhausting yourself at the start and not being able to get back.

I was soon trailing at the rear, but it's not a race. Gareth was running back and forth between the runners, who were quite spread out. After around ten minutes, I met a big, scary, tattooed man with two big, equally scary dogs. There was no one else in sight and I suddenly felt a bit vulnerable.
"You from the running club?" he said.
I mean, I was dressed in running gear and lots of other runners had just thundered past him, but given my speed I guess it was a valid question.
"Yes." there wasn't much else to say and he didn't look the type you wanted to upset.
"The local yobs keep putting things on the path to trip up runners. I come and clear them away a couple of times a week." Now I felt bad. Far from being scary, this man was actually the good guy.
"How long you been running?"
"About ten minutes. Five more and we will all turn round."
"No, I meant years."
"Oh! About six months."
"I think about running sometimes."
I didn't want to be rude, and I'm not physically built as a runner myself, but this guy really wasn't a runner's shape. Darts player maybe. But not running.

I gave him the club website details and explained couch to 5K. But I suspected it was just conversation he was making more than a serious running desire. Then I heard Gareth's whistle and it was time to turn round and head back.

At the next Couch to 5K, I went along to help and tattooed, scary man was there. He recognised me and we had a chat. He found the first session hard, but I recalled my own first session and advised him to do the homework runs and to stick with it.

He did stick with it. Sometimes the scary looking people are the nice people.

Another night at the club, the track was flooded after rain. So street running it was. There was a road loop which, I guess, was around a quarter of a mile long. We were going to do running and 'active rest' around it. Active rest basically means walking, but it keeps your heart working harder than stopping. Push yourself on the runs, keep active whilst resting.

The downside to the route is that it passes a chip shop. Each lap, the temptation got harder to resist. I wondered if I could pop in whilst passing one time and order, then pick them up passing the next time. I worked out I probably could, but my wallet was at the club and they'd be unlikely to set up a tab.

The trick to this circuit was ensuring you were close to the club when the final whistle went. If you are a quarter of the way round, you'd have to carry on for an extra lap. It's all about pace.

Many club members signed up to do the local 10K. Becky and Cath amongst them. Kristyan and I went to cheer them on. We waved them off at the start, then drove off to the top of the hill.

The route starts off with a hill climb. A punishing climb, a relentless climb. We stood at the top. Our reasoning was that they need the most encouragement then. Of course, the good news for the runners at that point is there's no more uphill after that.

We cheered and clapped. And as soon as they were out of site got back in the car and found another point to cheer and clap. And another. And another. Our brief was to keep them going, and we did well.

They completed the course and got their medals. Soon after that, Becky damaged her foot whilst running. Running can be a dangerous sport. My children and I preferred to run together so we left the club too. But we all took away happy memories and tremendous running tips.

19 ON YOUR BIKE

You may have noticed there is one exercise missing. Cycling. There's a reason for this.

When we had just two very small children, my then wife, Ruth, and I went for a drive out to the countryside. We ended up in the Manifold Valley. A former railway line, but now tarmacked, it's ideal for walking and cycling.

Although we didn't have a plan, it was June and the sun was out so we thought a walk might be nice. But on the car park was a bike hire kiosk. Neither of us had ridden a bike for many years. At least fifteen in my case.

We had a look at the bikes and the helpful assistant said how easy the trail was, how much fun it would be and we didn't need to hire them for a whole day; they would do a special four hour rate.

I explained I hadn't ridden one for at least fifteen years.
"You never forget how to ride a bike," he said. "Take one out for a ride round the car park to see."

I did, and it's true. I hadn't forgotten, I didn't fall off, I even managed a fairly straight line.

Back at the kiosk, they fitted a child seat to Ruth's bike for our eldest. Meanwhile, I had a trailer attached into which the car seat could be placed with the youngest still in it.

What a lovely family thing to do. We'd probably sign up to the National Trust and start shopping at Waitrose too. An idyllic family day out. Then we set off.

I think it's fair to say we knew it was going to be a disaster fairly early on. The eldest realised her only view was going to be of her mother's back and complained. But when Ruth turned round the bike would wobble. This did at least stop her complaining. However bad the view, it was better than a wobbling bike.

Meanwhile my trailer had a mind of its own and stubbornly refused to follow my bike, despite being attached. I'm fairly sure the wheels on it were made by the people who make supermarket trollies.

Of course, you already know that bike saddles are incredibly uncomfortable, but this was new to me. They make a hard, carved, church pew feel luxurious and soft. But why do they have to be so hard and so uncomfortable? There must a special place reserved in hell for the inventor of the bicycle saddle. Hopefully a particularly uncomfortable place.

After what was only a few yards, but felt like several miles, there was a tea shop. We agreed to stop there on the way back. We couldn't stop now as we knew we'd never get going again, and we had paid for four hours.

We bravely battled on. There was no shade and the sun was beating down on us. We hadn't planned to ride bikes so were simply not dressed for it.

Eventually I could stand the pain of the saddle no more, so got off and walked, pushing the bike. This was, of course, worse than walking as I had to push a bike.

Just four miles away the bike hirers had promised an ice cream shop. We'd easily get there and back in four hours they'd promised. I could walk there and back in four hours too. Just not if I was hampered by having to push the wretched bike I'd paid good money to hire.

Although not hurting my bottom, pushing the bike was painful in every other way imaginable. It also made me look like a wuss to everyone else. "Oh look at him," they'd all be saying to themselves, "can't even manage a four-mile bike ride. It's the children I feel sorry for. Loser." I couldn't bear the shame.

Back on the bike, I couldn't bear the pain. After a while, we did make it to an ice cream van. Never has anyone been so happy to have an ice cream. As an added bonus, there was some shade too. Ruth had to order the ice creams as I'd lost the power of speech some miles back. I was wet with sweat, smelled rank and was bright red. This called for a 99.

I lay on my back and offered up my body and soul. There were no takers. This meant only one thing; we were going to have to cycle back. I could have cried. Indeed, I would have cried, but I couldn't see how that would help the situation nor had I any fluid left in my body after all the sweating.

The journey back was no better. Indeed, it was worse. My bottom had gone through the pain to numb and back to pain again. But my legs were now also stiff and sore. My arms ached from having to pull the bike into line with the dodgy trailer and the sweat steamed up my glasses. I was having a miserable time.

We got back to the tea shop; we were over the four hours now, but we didn't even need to ask each other. We dismounted, threw the bikes to the ground and went in. There was quite a pile of discarded hire bikes from other foolish people like us. The tea shop was full of red-faced, sweaty people.

I can't tell you how comfortable the chairs were. I savoured every moment of a comfy seat. If ever cake was called for, this was the moment. I made it last as long as I could.

When we could drag it out no longer, we went back to the bikes. I couldn't face the pain of the saddle, so we pushed them back till we could see the hire kiosk. Then we hopped on and rode them back.

We were over an hour late. But I think they knew better than to argue about it. If my walk didn't say, "I can't sit down for a week now thanks to you," then the sweat and red face did. Or maybe the way we dumped the bikes down. They didn't charge us anyway.

And that is why I've never ridden a bike since.

20 SIMPLE SAILING

John Pantry has a song called 'Simple Sailing for Beginners.' Whilst sailing needs a sail, I only had a paddle, so tried paddling.

Whilst I was working in Devon, there was a firm that picked up holidaymakers in a minibus and took them paddling in a canoe down the Exe to the Turf Locks pub for a drink and bite to eat, before paddling back.

Having been recommending this to holidaymakers as an excellent fun thing, I thought maybe it was actually time to have a go at it. I'm not really a water person, so canoeing had never really been up there on my list of enjoyable things to do.

My lack of experience in such matters soon came to light when it turned out the canoes weren't canoes at all, but kayaks. I'd thought it was just a posh word for canoe.

The children were with me. The two eldest had their own kayaks, but the youngest had to share with me. But the only suitable one for that had two adult seats, so the instructor came with us in our boat too. This made me feel better.

We had to offload the kayaks from the minibus trailer and lower them into the water, whilst making sure they then didn't drift off before we'd got in them.

After a few minutes of paddling round in circles, the children eventually set off in a vaguely straight line. Meanwhile we headed off on a course straight as a die, not hitting the bank and keeping perfect rhythm. I think it's fair to say I wasn't doing the hard work in our boat.

The route really wasn't far but it took far longer by boat than walking. Or, more accurately, it took us much longer. To be fair, the children's route was much longer too as they zigzagged their way downstream. The instructor held our course straight, I didn't really bother paddling at all, I was only making it harder for him and he seemed to be managing perfectly well.

We got to the pub and scrambled out of the kayaks in a rather undignified manner. The key now was to ensure the boats were secured to something solid, so we didn't get back and find them drifting off to sea. Also, we had to make sure the paddles were secure and couldn't fall in the water. You don't want to be up the creek without a paddle.

We certainly looked the part at the pub as we had kept our life jackets on. We looked like the sporty family who had just paddled to the pub, probably from miles away and were going to go wild camping overnight. No point in spoiling the illusion by taking the life jackets off.

After we were suitably refreshed, we headed back to the kayaks. As far as I could make out, there was no dignified way to get back in. You either had to scramble around on the ground and try to slide across, or step in and hope it didn't capsize whilst you then tried to sit down.

Our kayaking skills hadn't improved any after the break. The children still zigzagged across the river crashing into one bank then the other. Meanwhile, the instructor effortlessly paddled us straight.

We got back to where the minibus was parked and the instructor glided our kayak up to the shore and jumped out. I scrambled about on the ground and lost any remaining dignity.

The children were pulled up against the shore excellently. It's just a shame it was the opposite bank. Eventually, they managed to paddle across the river.

All things considered, we decided water sports weren't for us. I was unconvinced John Pantry was right. There was no such thing as simple sailing: particularly for beginners.

21 HIGH IN THE SKY

The point of exercise, for a heart patient at least, is to get the heart working that little bit faster and that little bit harder. The heart is, after all, a muscle. All muscles are best when exercised. But you don't have to walk, run, swim, paddle or cycle. You can panic.

When we were on a family holiday, the holiday park had an aerial adventure. You were given a safety harness and a helmet, climbed up some stairs to treetop height, and then there was a series of obstacles to get over.

My heart started racing just climbing the stairs. The first obstacle was a series of hanging narrow planks, laid end to end but in a zigzag. Not too bad. Then came two wooden barrels laid sideways and end to end that you had to crawl through. The gap between them seemed minuscule from the ground, but when up there it was massive.

Then came a tightrope. There were ropes hanging down to hold onto so you were almost, but not quite, able to reach the next one whilst still holding onto the one before. I had a rope in my left hand, but however far I stretched, my right hand could not reach the next rope. I was stuck. I stood there high in the air for a few moments contemplating what to do.

There was an instructor on the ground below me.
"I'm stuck," I shouted down.
"Turn sideways," he shouted back.

Easier said than done when balancing on a wire at height. The wire started swinging precariously as I turned. But eventually I was sideways.

"Now slide your right foot out as far as you can and grab the rope with your right hand." This was easier from my new sideways position and I was underway again.

Next were hanging crosses. Each one independent of the others. This meant you could be swinging wildly on one and not be able to reach the next. To add to the sense of fun, you passed over the top of a tree too, just to add to the feeling of height.

Next were hanging tyres. Again, each one hanging independently, so a foot on each of two different ones left you doing the splits at height.

Then there was a vertical rope net. At least you had something to hold on to this time. The next obstacle was hanging wooden stepping-stones, again swinging individually. Then came the first zip wire.

It felt odd to hurl yourself off a platform with nothing to hold onto. I spent a few moments dithering about what to do, with helpful shouts from my children of "Just jump Dad."
I jumped. Swinging in the air is quite liberating. It was, of course, at this point that I realised the thing that was holding me on to the zip wire was the safety harness that held me on all the other obstacles. I was happy to trust it as a safety harness, just not on a zip wire. Once I'd realised the stupidity of this, I relaxed and enjoyed it. It felt good to glide through the air.

The course now disappeared into some woods, there was a net to walk along, some swinging planks, a tightrope and other obstacles interspersed with zip wires. In total eighteen obstacles to conquer.

A rope bridge brings you back out of the woods and you're faced with a staircase. You climb high up, the highest you've been on the course. This is the final zip wire descent. The wire stretches off into the distance, and the ground.

You jump off the platform and enjoy the ride. I even let go and flew down 'hands free.' You end up landing in a pile of wood chip. Here you disconnect your harness and walk back to the hut where you started.

When I started I was scared, but landing at the bottom of the last zip wire I was sorry it was over. It had been brilliant. A good heart workout too. But less exercise for my lungs and soles. Time to don the walking boots again.

22 MORECAMBE

Our next walk was unintentional. Well nearly anyway. Cath had attended teacher training college in Lancaster so we thought it would be nice to visit there and have a nosey around. But as the sea was close by, it seemed a shame not to visit the beach whilst so near. We found a leaflet of a walk from Lancaster to Morecambe. Maybe we could kill two birds with one stone.

In the end, we had no choice. We arrived at Lancaster station and found all the trains to Morecambe cancelled due to the staff being on strike. Why no one had thought to mention this when we purchased train tickets to Morecambe hours earlier, I don't know. Still, it solved our dilemma.

The only thing I knew about Lancaster is that it had a castle. I knew this because many years earlier my Aunt and Uncle had been in Lancaster and seen someone coming out of the castle.
"Can we go in?" they'd asked him.
"I've had lots of people asking if they can go out, but never anyone asking if they can go in," he replied.
Lancaster castle is a prison.

As we came out of Lancaster railway station, the walk leaflet directed us past the castle. I was surprised to see a sign saying it was open and you could go on a tour. It turns out it ceased being a prison in 2011

Although we didn't go on a tour as we had a coast to reach, we did have a look around the parts that are open without a tour. It was as you've seen on the TV series Porridge. An area of cells three stories high, safety nets between floors. Painted, what I imagine is called 'prison grey' on colour charts. Solid doors, no handles on the inside, a basic bed in each. No TV or en-suite. Those who say prison is a holiday camp would do well to have a visit. Can't say I'd fancy it. And I've been to Pontins.

At least the last prisoners here, however grim the conditions, were better off than previous inmates. Lancaster Castle has seen over 200 executions. It had also previously overseen witch trials. Its modern day uses include it being a licensed wedding venue.

You could embrace it all and get married, incarcerate the family and execute the in-laws, all in one venue. I'll let the marketing team know.

Our wedding plans secured, we carried on. The path fell steeply. Lancaster really is quite hilly. Cath pointed out various buildings on distant hilltops that were part of the college, recounting what each one was from her memory.

We were down by the river now. The main railway line crossing over it at ninety degrees. But branching off was an old railway line, now a walkway, to Morecambe. Trains currently take around ten minutes, when they're running; we took around an hour and a half to walk it. Still, we got to see Lancaster. The path passes an ASDA and we stopped off for a drink and the toilet. We carried ever onwards.

At one point the path crosses the railway line. As the sign instructed us to do, we stopped, looked and listened. There were no trains, which we already knew. Once safely over the tracks there was an unusual sight ahead. A lady, I'd guess in her late thirties, dressed as if it was the 1950s, pushing an old-fashioned bicycle.

I'd never understood why people pushed bikes until my bike riding experience. Now she had my full sympathy. But why did she have a bike? And why was she dressed from seventy years ago? As

walkers do, she smiled and said,
"Hello." as we passed her.
"Hello," we replied. Too polite to ask why.

Not long after, we arrived in Morecambe. There was a man and his wife arm in arm, dressed in Victorian outfits. Is Morecambe in some kind of time warp? We went to the sea front. There were a couple of people in 1920s outfits.

I looked around; most people were in period costume of one sort or another. This could be normal behaviour in Morecambe, I don't know. They may be eyeing my mobile phone as some sort of witchcraft. I daren't try to explain electricity to them.

We strolled along the front, looking the odd ones out in our 21st century jeans and t- shirts. Then we saw the sign. "Welcome to Morecambe Vintage By The Sea Festival." They clearly take their events seriously in Morecambe. But at least it explained it.

It was actually quite brilliant. There were coconut shies and other old-fashioned games and rides. There was an old art deco mobile cinema; an original vehicle lovingly restored and showing original pathe news clips about Morecambe, along with a short film about its own history and restoration.

There were vintage bus rides down the sea front to Happy Mount Park, where we played a round of pirate themed crazy golf, before getting a vintage bus back. I couldn't have been happier. Well, I could; there were still no trains back to Lancaster. I really didn't fancy the four mile walk back.

We found the bus station in Morecambe. It was on the dual carriageway near the railway station. As if to mock the railways, there were lots of buses running. Checking the timetable, it took the bus about an hour. I knew it would be longer than the train, but I couldn't understand why so much longer. The answer soon became apparent. We toured, at a guess, every street in Morecambe, before arriving back on the dual carriageway opposite the bus station twenty-five minutes later. This time we set off in the direction of Lancaster and we even recognised some of the route from our walk. The bus even pulled into ASDA.

Eventually the bus made it to Lancaster bus station. Wearily, we realised this was at the bottom of the hill, whereas the railway station was at the top. We made it to the station just in time for the train. It's just a shame the train didn't; it was delayed. Public transport hadn't been our friend today. But everything else had.

In fairness to Britain's railways, when I contacted the train company who sold us the tickets and asked them why they had sold them, knowing there were no trains, they said as it was the company who cancelled the trains that had delayed our journey, they should pay us compensation and to contact them.

I did. They said, as we'd abandoned our journey, the company who sold us the tickets should refund them and I should contact them.

I did. They said…well you get the idea. Eventually, I said to both of them what the other had said and, in a surprise move, they both came back and said,
"It's not really our fault, the other company should pay, but as a gesture of goodwill we will pay you the full cost of the return travel tickets."
I'd not only had a free day out; I'd made a profit on it.

And they say Britain's railways are incompetently run.

23 TO THE MANOR BORN

Many, many years ago, there was a local stately home that rarely opened its doors. Occasionally its gardens, but never its doors. One day, probably for some special occasion, but it was over thirty years ago so I can't remember, the family announced they were going to open it up for a day.

My mum, and her friends, wanted to go and I was duly designated driver. Going round large houses is all well and good, and I'll stare appreciatively at antiques and portraits, but without ever knowing what it is, exactly, I'm expected to appreciate. So it's largely wasted on me.

When we arrived, there was a young lady in the hall taking admission fees. As we were roughly the same age, and no one else was, we fell into conversation. I had noticed she was rather pretty too. It turned out she was a daughter of the owner. It was time to work my charm. If I married into it and lived in the house, I was sure I'd learn to appreciate it all.

It turned out a new portrait of her brother had just been unveiled. He had an improbably posh name like Bartholomew or some such. The sort of name that would get you beaten up at a comprehensive school anyway.

Unbelievable though it may seem, the daughter was impervious to my charms, and I never did marry into life in a stately home.

Now, over thirty years later, I was recounting this story to Cath as we drove up the house drive. The first time I'd been back. The gardens and house are now regularly open; times change, and clearly they need the revenue. Don't we all.

As we approached the top of the drive, there was a wooden hut with a man sat in it. He was taking admission fees. He asked if we'd been before.

"Once, many years ago," I said. "The hall was open and I was chatting to one of the daughters." I smiled at the memory, "There was a new portrait of her brother. Bartholomew or something."

"Ah," he chuckled. "That'll be me. The portrait is in storage now though. It's no longer new."

I was just grateful I hadn't said anymore about his sister. That could have been embarrassing.

We parked up. Although small by stately home standards, there were plenty of grounds to explore. So explore we did. Bartholomew had given us a map. I can't imagine living somewhere that needs a map. I wonder where his sister lives.

There was a path down to a lake. I've known houses to have a pond, but this was a lake. It had a boat house and an island. You couldn't take a boat out onto the lake, nor could you walk round it, as the gardens gave way to arable land, but it was still part of the estate.

There was a woodland you could explore. Someone had placed wicker animal shapes at strategic points, so when you looked into the distance, for a moment, at first glance, they looked like real animals.

After we'd explored that, there was an area probably best described as informal garden. In this area was what the map called the dog graveyard. We found the headstones of the former family dogs. One was, apparently, called Pussy. Either that dog had an identity crisis, or they'd opened it up to other pets too. Mind you,

Pussy does lack imagination for a name if it's your pet cat.

We then strolled round the formal garden area closest to the house. Off this was a walkway, along which they grew fifty varieties of snowdrops. Forty-nine more than I knew existed. Some were clearly different. Others you felt someone was having a laugh. You know when you get a paint catalogue and there's a page of beige where someone has come up with fifty different names for beige, but they're all the same colour? That's what had happened here with the snowdrops. It's not so much the snowdrops were different, just the names for them.

Next, it was into the walled vegetable garden. Part of the wall is formed by the Head Gardeners cottage, and still lived in to this day by the Head Gardener. Of course, his duties have changed over the years. He's no longer responsible for all the young garden boys who used to live in one hut in another corner of the walled garden. They also had to keep the fires burning that heated the greenhouses.

The other claim to fame here, is that the current Head Gardener holds the world record for the largest gooseberry. It was the size of an egg.

We ambled over to one of the farm buildings. It was staging an art sale. Local artists had work on display. There were some excellent works, some more abstract pieces, and some which, quite frankly, I could have done better myself. With my eyes shut. I can appreciate a good painting. But I also know a shoddy bit of work when I see one.

However, my interest was the homemade cakes. It was unclear whose home they were made in, but it did say 'home made' so it must have been someones. I had a piece of flapjack. Oats are good for your heart. Admittedly, syrup and sugar are less good. But focus on the positives.

As we drove out of the drive, the church opposite the exit had a flower festival on. It promised free admission, so we parked up and went in. We were greeted by an enthusiastic volunteer who certainly gave the impression that he had been waiting all day for us to turn up and that now we were here, his life was complete.

He gave us a laminated card with a history of the church on, and a plan of the interior highlighting the important things to look for. As we set off for the stained-glass window, he greeted the next arrivals with the same enthusiasm.

The church was beautifully decorated. Flowers were arranged everywhere and they'd clearly gone to a lot of effort. I settled down to read the lengthy history information on the card. The history is easily told. An earlier Bartholomew (the family had a distinct lack of imagination when naming their children) had wanted a church to worship in, as travelling to a neighbouring village to worship was, quite frankly, tedious. Particularly on a Sunday when there were no buses. So, in 1861 he commissioned someone to build this church.

Bartholomew died during its construction, so his son Bartholomew saw it through. Even then, builders were over ambitious with estimates, and there was a problem when the builder couldn't afford to pay his workers. So Bartholomew stepped in and paid for him. Apparently, the current Bartholomew still worships there now.

24 TAKING A BATH

Having visited Cath's old alma mater, it was time for a stroll round mine. I didn't go to university, but I did go to boarding school. Long before Harry Potter made it popular. The school is located in the Roman city of Bath, although the Romans called it Aquae Sulis. Which is Latin for Bath.

They say that, like Rome, Bath is built on seven hills. But I haven't counted them and don't know anyone who has. I guess that's what they hope for. You can say what you like if you know no one will check.

Driving in, the road from the motorway takes you past the school before you get to the city. Actually, the road takes you past the school playing fields before the school. I was never a sports fanatic. I find watching it as boring as playing it. But twice a week we were forced up here for games. Monday and Wednesday afternoons.

Autumn term was rugby. This was far and away the worst. It struck me as an unnecessarily violent game. Although this seemed to be the appeal to some of the staff. It was also the coldest term of course. The playing fields were a bleak spot for an eleven-year old boy. Turns out they're a bleak spot for a fifty-year old man too. The trees were all angled from the wind. One teacher used to delight in telling us there was nothing between us and Siberia. Certainly it was cold enough to believe, but I couldn't check then as we didn't have the internet.

The spring term gave rise to hockey. This was certainly more bearable. But after they abandoned the bully-off, the appeal dwindled. I found it easier to avoid the ball in hockey. This was my sole purpose in sport; avoid any contact with the ball. Some staff couldn't grasp the concept of not liking sport. They kept trying to get us (there were several of us who had no interest in it) to join in. Occasionally, they would make me be captain. The only difference this made, was that I wasn't last to be picked.

In the Summer term we did, in theory at least, get a choice. There was tennis, athletics or cricket. In reality, only those good at tennis or athletics got to do those. The rest of us played cricket. This suited us. Even a fully involved, enthusiastic player of cricket spends most of the time standing round chatting. If I was on the batting side, I'd be so far down the batting list that I never needed to worry about putting pads on, as the time would run out before I'd be in. When fielding, I knew the best spots to pick where the ball never went. Cricket suited me fine.

Although rugby was played regardless of the weather, hockey and cricket weren't played in bad weather. Instead, they were replaced with the dreaded cross-country run. The route seemed to encompass all of Bath's seven uphills.

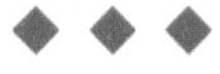

I had emailed ahead to ask if it was ok to visit and been assured it was and someone would meet us at 1 o'clock. I'd asked if we could join in the school lunch as there were lessons on Saturday morning. I was told that there are no longer Saturday lessons and therefore no Saturday school lunch. Youngsters don't know how lucky they are these days.

As it was morning, and we were passing the school anyway, we parked there and caught the bus down to the city. Memories came flooding back of Thursday and Saturday afternoons. To make up for having lessons on a Saturday morning, we had Thursday afternoons off.

We got off the bus in Bath city centre. We went to the Abbey. They were doing major renovation work and large parts of it were cordoned off. But we could still get a feel for the place.

We walked up to The Circus. This is a large circle of townhouses. There are three entrances to the circle and each one faces houses so you always see houses when entering. The central area is laid to lawn. It looks very posh. I imagine the residents get little peace though. Crowds of tourists pour through it.

We had a look at the actual Roman Baths, but one look at the admission price was enough to dissuade us from going in. Anyway, we had to get back to school. We hopped back onto the bus.

We were met at the main school entrance by our guide. This in itself felt like a treat; as pupils we were not allowed to use this entrance. This was the posh area. Invited guests and visitors only. Part of me had expected the whole school to be in a 1980s time warp. Everything going on unchanged from when I left. But the discovery that Saturday morning lessons were no longer a thing, put paid to that.

Of course, many buildings remained unaltered. The classrooms were as I left them. There may even have been some of my work still on the wall. The dining hall too was identical, all as I remembered it. But other things had changed of course. No need for the pay phone anymore of course. No one could imagine a mobile phone when I was at school.

We had one computer for the whole school, and it was really little more than an oversized calculator. It took up most of the room. But even then, we knew computers were the way forward. Although we never imagined we'd one day have our own at home. Less still in the palm of our hands.

The dormitories were no more. Instead, accommodation was in new purpose-built buildings. Not dissimilar to a travelodge.

Times change of course. When I was there, most pupils were boarders; now there are so few there are no Saturday lessons. The few boarders now are all foreign students. They expect a high standard. They get it.

When I was still a pupil, they built a new sports hall. It's still there and in use, but of course rather dated now. They want to update it all. Make a multipurpose hall. The hall we used is now the library. The library a computer suite. I guess the days of the library are numbered. Books are old technology.

Sugar is the current evil, so the tuck shop is gone. Now it's a day area for day pupils. But they can't buy aniseed balls, crisps, or cans of pop. We needed the E numbers for all the exercise we had to do. The modern pupils must be exhausted. Kale and rice cakes may be better for you, but you don't get the energy boost.

As we walked around the grounds and between the various buildings, it did strike me how fit we had to be. Dashing between lessons, back to dormitories and day rooms, up to the playing fields. We'd completed several miles this afternoon and done nowhere near a school day.

Having seen it all and relived memories from my childhood, we set off home. But we decided to buy supplies for the return trip so popped back down to the city. We found a Sainsbury's. The car park was on the original railway station and the original station canopies formed covered parking.

We strolled down to the river and ate some sandwiches near the current railway station. Bath is quite a compact city, and it's very lovely. I don't think I appreciated it fully when I was at school. But then why would I.

They say you never forget a good teacher, so I should probably pay homage to Mr Lewis. He inspired my love of writing and the ability to make a story out of anything. Everything can be fun if you look at it the right way. Enjoy what you do, enjoy what you see, enjoy writing about it. He was, of course, my Biology teacher.

I know Biology isn't the first subject that springs to mind when you consider writing stories, but that was Mr Lewis' ability. He saw your strengths and played to them. I remember writing a story on "The history of soil." He was so impressed, I got 50p to spend in the tuck shop. Enough for a quarter of strawberry bon bons, ten aniseed balls, a bag of crisps and a can of Coke. Of course, I'm hopeless at Biology, but hopefully the fact you've read this far, means I'm good at writing stories.

Of course, he wasn't everyone's favourite teacher. The fact his nickname was 'Hitler' was a clue to him being rather strict. At the start of your first lesson with him, he would get you to write his 'standard line' inside the back cover of your exercise book. "Few things are more distressing to a well- regulated mind, than to see a child, who ought to know better, disporting themselves at im-proper moments." The first thing you notice about the 'standard line' is that it's more than a line long, which made writing it out several times tedious. So I'm told.

But it's Mr Lewis you need to thank, or curse, that this book exists at all.

25 SUPER WEST

The closest seaside to Bath is Weston Super Mare. I knew it had the nickname Weston Super Mud, but I'd never been. Cath and I went there for our next exercise.

Once we arrived at the beach, it was lovely and sandy. I thought its nickname was a bit unfair. We strolled down the front. It was a red, hot sunny day. The beach was already filling up. There wasn't much space on the sand, but the water was empty. There were donkey rides and even donkeys pulling carriages you could ride in on the beach. Some of the carriages were made to look like Thomas The Tank Engine. Someone clearly hadn't thought this through. If Thomas is, as his name suggests, an engine, then he doesn't need to be pulled by a horse.

Back on the sea front, there was a crazy golf course with an aerial adventure overhead. But they wanted £7 each just for a game of crazy golf. I like a game. But not that much.

Further down, we found another crazy golf course. £2 each. Bargain. It was slightly older and a little faded, but perfectly playable. When walking, it's advisable to get some sport in too.

Walking by the sea is always more agreeable than walking around a town, or even in the countryside, I find. Countryside is very nice, but there's something even nicer about the beach. Out to sea, there was a large island visible from the main sea front and a smaller island which you can only see once you've walked much further round. The smaller one had an old pier out to it, but this was rusted, decaying and dangerous. Which was a shame, as it's the only pier in the country to go to an island.

It's fenced off to stop any intrepid explorers going down it anyway. The locals want it restored to its former glory. Or restored to a useable condition at the very least. But the company that own it want to build a new hotel first, on land near the pier, and many fear they'll never do the pier. The locals are fundraising to buy it and restore it themselves.

This might seem ambitious, but they cite nearby Clifton, where locals salvaged their pier and restored it. It's won awards now apparently. "Best Pier in Clifton" is possibly one. We knew all this as there was a group of people at the fenced off entrance explaining their hopes and dreams. And naturally asking for our financial support.

Weston does have a pier, but you have to pay to go on and that sort of thing annoys me, so we didn't. They still want to relieve you of more money once you're on it, but they're not fleecing me twice. However, it did look nice from the shore.

If they do restore the other pier, I hope it's free to go on. After our impromptu chat, we had missed the open top bus back so all we could do was walk back, following its tail lights into the distance.

Whilst we'd been gone, the tide had gone out, and it was now clear how the town got its nickname. Where the sea had been before, was now mud. There was still the sand, but it now went to mud, then to sea. I could see why no one was in the water.

Further the other way, on the part of the beach the tide never gets to, was a sand sculpture exhibit. I am always impressed with these things, as I struggle to make sandcastles with the children. But time was against us and we didn't have chance to go. We had to make do with the bits peeking over the top of the fence. We had time for an ice cream to cool down though.

We did holiday in Weymouth however, where they also have sand sculptures.

26 IT'S IN THE SAND

Apparently, the sand of Weymouth is perfect for building sand-castles. Scientists have been out with their buckets and spades and concluded that the texture of the sand is perfect for building. Fred Darrington took it one step further and created sand sculptures.

That was over ninety years ago and now his grandson Mark runs Sandworld. But they still have sand sculptures on the beach for you to admire. Indeed, this was the first I knew about Weymouth's sand building quality.

There's a covered area on the beach, which you can see from the promenade, which shows them off. Naturally, there's information about Sandworld too. I knew the children would love it. And I knew I would too.

Most of Sandworld is under a marquee to protect the sculptures from wind and rain. They are made solely from sand and water. Some have colours added for artistic effect. For example, the 'Finding Nemo' scene had Nemo coloured in orange, white and black. It made the sculpture even more striking.

We spent a surprising amount of time looking round them. And then went round a few more times, spotting different details each time. Then we went to build our own.

There's basically a large sand pit with hoses and tubes and buckets to fill with sand and make the biggest structure you can. There are staff on hand to help get the right consistency of sand and water. That, it turns out, is crucial. Once you have it right, you can turn out an impressively tall tower and carve large chunks out of it. The key, of course, is to stop before it collapses.

Nearby is a pirate themed crazy golf course. I don't know why so many crazy golf courses are pirate themed; maybe pirates weren't as bad as they are made out to be and enjoyed a round of crazy golf. Although I'd think playing it on board a ship was an added obstacle.

There was a little train running round a park, and also a fitness trail. Be rude not to. Every so often on the lap round the park there was an exercise board with instructions on what to do.

We walked back onto the sea front and down to the main area. They even have a crazy golf course on the beach. If you're thinking of visiting a British seaside, an interest in crazy golf certainly helps.

When I was eight or nine we went on holiday to Jersey. Given that I'd never been abroad, this was a big event. We sailed from Weymouth. I know they drive on the left, use sterling, have the Queen's head on their stamps and all things British, but it was across the water. That made it abroad in my book.

Although it was summer, it was dark when we arrived at Weymouth as we were on the overnight sailing. I don't remember how we got to the ferry terminal, but I guess we got a taxi. I do remember not overly enjoying being in a cabin in the depths of the ship. I don't think I slept much. I don't think I let the others sleep much either.

I do remember going out on deck the next morning and seeing nothing but sea all around me. Eventually, Jersey appeared in the distance. The ship appeared to go painfully slowly. The return journey was a daytime sailing; it lasted hours but felt like days. As the ships got larger, they could no longer leave from Weymouth, and that was the end of Weymouth as a ferry port.

So I was surprised to see a massive ship moored at the port. It turns out, full circle, ships could now dock again and the Channel Islands were back in reach of Weymouth. Just like the Exmouth ferry leaving from Starcross railway station, so the Jersey ferry left from a railway station too. Although this ferry was massive and the station tiny. And shut.

There's a railway line just next to Weymouth railway station. You can't see it as it's overgrown with weeds. It crosses the road then runs down a side street and continues all the way down the road to the harbour station. The harbour station has trains on one side of the platform and ships on the other. It could not be handier.

Of course, given the fact it runs down a street, it makes operating trains slightly tricky, and slow. When the ferries stopped, naturally enough the trains stopped. When the ferries restarted, the train companies pretended not to notice and the tracks sit in the road rusting and being a nuisance to cyclists. There are calls to have them taken out (the tracks, not the cyclists) but there are counter calls to use them again.

The railway line from the ferry, and therefore the road, follows the side of a small waterway up to a marina near the station. The only way across, at first glance, is by a road bridge some way up the road. Trains can just fit under it on the track but sailing boats with masts can't. Therefore it is a lifting bridge, and several times a day the road closes when the bridge is lifted.

But there is another way across the water for pedestrians. You can be rowed across. It's not expensive and the rowing ferry has been in existence since the 16th Century. The old man who took us across looked like he'd been doing since the opening day. I wanted to say, "You take it easy, I'll do it for you." But part of me thought that it might, despite my best intentions, come across as rude. It also looked very hard work. It would be embarrassing to tell an old man he was working too hard, then not be able to do it myself. I just sat back and enjoyed the very short ride. We walked back on the other side to the lifting bridge. A few yachts were waiting to pass under. The road duly closed, the bridge raised and the boats moved under. It was quite satisfying to watch.

27 SOMETHING STRANGE IN THE AYR

The Scottish are very proud of Robert Burns. He's regarded as their national poet. There's even a Burns day when they pipe in a haggis and recite his poem about haggis. Yes, he wrote a poem about haggis. He's also credited with Auld Lang Syne, but he actually adapted it from a traditional folk song.

The house where he was born and lived with his six siblings and parents is open to visitors and laid out as it would have been when he was there. I think it's fair to say it was cosy, although I'd have made the gift shop into another bedroom.

You can wander around the gardens too. They aren't big, and across the road is the Robert Burns museum. The fact they have made a whole museum about him, shows the respect they hold him in.

My interest in being in Ayr though was not Burns related. It was to do with the electric brae. Brae, in Scotland, means hill or slope. Electric comes from when they thought magical forces were at play. You see, when you arrive at the brae from Ayr, it appears to be just like any other road heading downhill. Except if you stop the car on this one, it rolls back uphill.
"This isn't possible, you cry, and, of course, it's not. Hence why they thought magical forces were at play. It's really strange and were it anywhere else would probably need some kind of traffic system in place. But being in a remote corner of Scotland, there's

rarely more than two cars there.

Halfway 'down' there's a small lay-by and a plaque which gives a very brief history. We parked the car and had come prepared. We got out a ball; it rolled uphill. We poured water out of a bottle; it flowed uphill. We got back in the car; it was a massive hefty car. I'd ordered a small one from the hire company but they'd sent this massive thing instead. I took the handbrake off; it rolled uphill.

The children were amazed. I was amazed. It was amazing. As we stood on the roadside marvelling at this spectacle, a cyclist came by, having to pedal really hard to get downhill. A couple more came by the other way, freewheeling uphill.

Another family turned up. They'd brought a skateboard. The youngest set off rolling uphill. They were amazed.

There's a small stream by the roadside; it flowed uphill.

I knew the answer to this riddle and yet even standing there, I couldn't fathom how it might be. Like a good conjurer performing a trick, the effect is amazing and the explanation is very simple. It's all an optical illusion.

The surrounding hills, apparently, distort your view. Your brain takes in the information and the only way it can make sense is to reverse the hill. Your brain goes along with it. So what you see is the opposite of what is real. Even armed with this information, I couldn't see how it was possible.

We got in the car and carried on to Culzean Castle. It's a National Trust property and is everything you'd expect. There's a house, formal gardens and a woodland to explore. We did it all and walked miles and made the most of the weather. But I had an ulterior motive. I'd been told that from Culzean Castle you could see the Electric Brae and from the angle of view there, the hills made sense and the magic was revealed.

You could indeed see the Electric Brae. But it still looked opposite to me. What had seemed uphill there, was still uphill from here. As optical illusions go, this has to be the best.

We drove back, this time cruising uphill. Cars coming the other way continued to stop and roll back uphill. The locals are used to it and are very patient.

When we got home, I did further research. I found a video online. They pointed a camera out towards the sea and drew a line across the horizon. When the camera swung inland, the line stayed on the screen, and it clearly showed the Electric Brae was, indeed, an optical illusion. The problem is, when you're on it you can't see the horizon.

28 THE TWO SAINTS

There's a long-distance footpath from Lichfield to Chester. A traditional pilgrimage route of ninety-two miles. Cath had wanted to do it, so I bought her the guidebook. It turned out she wanted me to do it with her too.

So, one Sunday afternoon we gathered up a handful of our children and set off. Obviously, we weren't going to do the full ninety-two miles, we're not stupid. But we did the first section from Lichfield, just six miles.

Planning ahead is key so we parked one car at our intended finish point, then drove in the other car to Lichfield to begin.

The two saints in question are St Chad and St Werburgh. St Chad used to prefer travel by foot rather than horseback as it meant he could meet and talk to more people. He used to stand in his well and pray, and it was also the sight of his many miracles. Thus people used to flock to see him and so Lichfield Cathedral was built.

St Werburgh on the other hand was, by all accounts, a bit of a looker. She had advances off many men, but shunned them all to open convents instead. She's buried at Chester Cathedral.

Walks are very flexible, so you can go either way. Lichfield to Chester is St Chad's Way. Chester to Lichfield is St Werburgh's Way. We were following St Chad.

The walk starts at St Chad's Well. The one he stood in to pray.

It then passes Lichfield Cathedral and through town. We had the guidebook but we were promised waymarkers too. We hadn't seen one so far. Clearly, you had to buy the guidebook to do the walk; a cunning marketing ploy there.

Randomly, we then spotted our first one; it was a nice reassurance. We followed it down a country lane. On the right was an old cave where they used to sell candles to pilgrims walking to Chester. I can't see they'd make much money doing that today. And how many candles would you need?

The walk continues across fields. Often with waymarkers, and equally often without. We came up with a new game. We all guessed how many waymarkers we would see. I said eight, Cath said ten and the children went for seventeen and twenty-seven. So far we were on two.

As the path ventured further into the countryside, there were more of them, but without the guidebook you'd be hard pressed to follow the route. Memories of the Heritage Trail came flooding back. Particularly when we emerged out of the field onto a road that the guidebook failed to mention and with no waymarkers.

We retraced our steps before finding an alternative, not waymarked, path. We followed it and it duly brought us to a waymarker randomly in the middle of a field. We carried on, buoyed by its presence.

Then we came to another choice. There was a waymarker, but the route it wanted you to take was less than clear. It could have been either. The guidebook wasn't overly clear. We sent smallest child up ahead to see. He scampered off and gave us a big thumbs up from the far end of the field.

We carried on, waymarkers and book working in harmony for a while. The route now followed a quiet country lane, before disappearing down a path in some woodland. We carried on and the path became quite muddy. Then muddier still. Eventually, we ended up having to balance our way along a fallen branch.

The path dried out a little and the woodland opened up on our left. Suddenly there was a post in the path and a waymarker telling us to go left and uphill. At the top of the hill, we were rewarded with a view across fields and in the distance, Lichfield Cathedral. It looked a long way off. I wouldn't want to be doing the walk the other way and see that I still had all that left to walk.

Less than two miles for us to go now. We came out onto some heath land, then passed a reservoir and came out onto a road. We walked down the road and saw our final waymarker of the day, number twenty-four, pointing into the car park. Just eighty-seven miles left to Chester.

We got in the car, drove back to Lichfield for the other car, and headed home. It's a lovely feeling when you get home from a long walk.

29 I'LL HAVE THE SAME PLEASE

There are many ways to wake up in the morning. My favourite is to get a text from Cath saying she's in an ambulance with sirens blaring and blue lights flashing, on her way to hospital. Sadly, she let me down. And simply texted that she'd woken up with palpitations in the night and felt giddy and lightheaded in the shower that morning. I did what any boyfriend would do in that situation. Told her to get a grip and not to forget to get something for my tea.

For reasons I can't imagine, she ignored my advice and called the NHS instead. Once she told them what was wrong with her, they dispatched an ambulance. They duly arrived. As I wasn't there, I don't know the actual conversation that took place, but it appeared to be along the lines of,
"You may want to take your phone charger with you, so you can charge your phone."
"Should I take my shoes?"
"No, no need for them, slippers are fine."
"Coat?"
"No, just make sure you have your phone charger."
Just to ensure they could justify this advice, they then encouraged her to ring everyone from the back of the ambulance. She rang into work, she called me. I'm not saying it wasn't critical to get her to hospital as quickly as possibly, but I'm just saying I'm sure they only used the sirens when they knew she was on the

phone. It certainly added dramatic effect.

Due to geographical distances, my arrival at hospital was only shortly after hers. And I didn't have blue lights or sirens. And I had to park the car. You can't put a price on health, but they have a good go at it in the car park.

I then arrived at A&E reception. It's hard to imagine a more soulless and depressing place. It's not as good when you're not the patient. The receptionists are sat behind reinforced glass panels, meaning all medical and intimate details have to be shouted across. It does make for a fun game though, as you try to work out who the person shouting through the glass is with. All of them appeared to be sitting comfortably, so the shouted symptoms didn't match. But then someone shuffled out of the toilet, and we all knew what was up with them.

Soon it was my turn to shout across the counter. Being deaf, I had the added disadvantage of not knowing what was being shouted back at me. And thus the waiting room was treated to watching a receptionist screaming at full volume "THROUGH THE DOUBLE DOORS AND TO THE AMBULANCE CORRIDOR" At first, I thought a corridor was an odd place to keep ambulances. But it turns out it's simply where they keep the patients who arrived by ambulance. A brand new multi-million-pound hospital, and it had apparently occurred to no one that ambulances need to put patients somewhere when they arrive. So corridor it is.

But first, I needed to get through the double doors. I guess it's security, but the double doors were electronically locked. With no obvious way through, it was just a matter of hanging around till a staff member showed up with an electronic key fob. Sure enough, a nurse soon came along and thankfully I knew the secret password, "Can I come in?" And that was it. I was in. Thank goodness for tight security; you wouldn't want just anyone being able to get access.

By this time, she was out of the corridor and into a bay, but only just, and I could see her feet-resplendent in slippers-sticking out. As always when you arrive in hospital, there is a flurry of activity. Wires here, drips there and the machine that goes "beep." Turns out the machine shouldn't go "beep" at all. It was only doing it constantly because her heart was racing along at 170; at rest it should be 50.

They started a drip, and this had the effect of making her feel ill, and not reducing the heart rate. The Dr then said there was a choice; they could either pump her full of a different medicine, or put her to sleep, wire her up to the mains and give her an electric shock. That sounded fun to me, but she chose the medication.

They started the new drip and all was going well. On the second bag of drip, they sat her up, brought her some cardboard, which they optimistically called sandwiches, and she promptly felt really ill. The colour (such as it was) drained from her, she became cold yet sweaty and doctors and nurses appeared from all directions.

The drip was taken off, and I was given the job of holding it with my thumb on the end of the tube. Meanwhile, they tilted the bed to make her head lower than the rest of her and struck up conversation to keep her awake.
"What do you do?"
"I'm a teacher...I teach."
"Oh. I've got children."
"I teach children."
And it's this high brow conversation that keeps patients awake and alive. But it was a bit too intellectual for me, so I didn't join in. It took all my concentration not to take my thumb off the tube.

It turned out they were a little over-enthusiastic with the drip and her heart rate was now too low! But nature kicked in and restored balance and her heart settled into its regular rhythm. Once recovered, she was relieved and the doctor disappointed, as he thought it wouldn't work and was desperate to do the electrocution. Although he called it something else that sounded slightly less dangerous.

After that, she slept for several hours. It's considered acceptable for patients to sleep but not really for their visitors. But equally there's not much to do. I played with the buttons on the bed for a bit but that nearly woke her up a few times. In the end I went for a walk, carefully remembering the route so I could get back. Left at the man with the swollen foot, right at the old lady, and through the doors by the person who was ahead of me at reception when I got there, and was now lying face down.

Once Cath had woken and managed to eat, she was discharged, with strict instructions to take it easy, avoid alcohol, fizzy drinks and stress. She manages the first three very well anyway. Her white blood cell count was also low. Apparently, this makes you tired. Iron makes it higher, so I told her to do more ironing.

As she came in her slippers, she now had to walk out in her slippers. This did rather look like she'd escaped as she wandered the streets in her slippers. I guess I should have given her a lift, but I told her where the bus stop was.

Taking it easy apparently means being unable to cook tea, but fortunately I was on hand to help there. After my home-cooked meal, she decided maybe she could cook in future to build herself up.

The doctor's advice was, "take a few days off work till you feel better. If it happens again call an ambulance." Then, with a glint in his eye, "We can always try the electrical charge then." Maybe that's his way to make sure you don't come back.

30 AWARD WINNING

We were in Salford in Manchester. The children and I had come for a tour of the BBC studios. Except, of course, they also film ITV and Channel 4 programmes there too.

We saw the actual BBC Sports studio. We saw how they film Newsround and the CBBC continuity desk. We saw TV studios; we saw radio studios.

In the radio studio they had a flight of stairs with five different floor coverings on each step, to make different noises. They had a small kitchen with various appliances. Apparently, radio audiences can tell the difference in noise between hot water and cold water being poured out of a kettle. We had to shut our eyes and see if we could. I couldn't, but a surprising number of people in the group could.

The highlight though was the Blue Peter studio. The actual Blue Peter studio. We got to stand behind the doors all the celebrities enter through. It's basically just a large cupboard. We got to sit where the presenters sit. We got to walk across the hallowed Blue Peter floor. The studio is surprisingly small; to make it look larger on TV the presenters have to take, what are called in the trade, 'presenter steps.' These are small steps but more of them. The aim is to make it look like they are taking more steps to give the impression that the studio is larger.

They then showed us the Blue Peter badges. You may feel there is only one badge, but no, there are various different ones.

When I was around six years old, I drew a monster and sent it in for a competition. I won. The only time in history my artwork has won an award. I got a white round badge with a blue Blue Peter ship on it and the words "competition winner" written round the edge. I couldn't have been more thrilled.

Since 2005, these badges have been replaced by the standard shield shape badge, but with an orange background instead of white. But still the blue ship.

There is, of course, the standard shield shape with a white background and blue ship. These are worn by the presenters and are also given to viewers who appear on the show, or to a viewer who writes in with an interesting story.

If you already have one of those and go on to make another achievement you get a silver ship on a blue shield.

There are also green, purple and special anniversary editions.

The only other one is the gold badge. Essentially, for this you have to achieve something outstanding. Saving someone's life or inventing a new vaccine are generally accepted reasons. Presenters are given one on their last show, and whilst I'm not one to knock that achievement, I'm not sure it's gold badge worthy.

When we got home, my daughter wrote to Blue Peter and explained about my heart attack and that she looked after me when I came out of hospital. She got a letter back with a Blue Peter badge. They also felt I deserved something, but apart from the gold badge you have to be under 18 to get a Blue Peter badge. Or a presenter. So they sent me a cloth badge. I was thrilled all over again.

Cath's sister's husband, Christie Spurling, got an MBE off the Queen. All well and good, but it's not a Blue Peter badge is it? And he's only got one MBE. I've got two Blue Peter badges.

You can read Christie's story at

https://www.n-gage.org.uk/story/the-team/

ACKNOWLEDGEMENT

So many people were involved in this book that to name any does seem a bit unfair on the others. To everyone who was involved, a big thank you. But special thanks must go to Martha for her enthusiasm for the project and endless help getting it together, particularly the technical side of it. To Jo for the inspiration for the cover design (check out her work at Jo Spurling Art) and her general enthusiasm. To my children for coming on walks with me when they'd rather be at home: or anywhere else at all. To Tracy, Ruth, Kristyan and Becky, without whom I wouldn't be here to tell the story in the first place. And on that subject, all the NHS staff and everyone at the BHF. These people work tirelessly and their only reward is to spend time with me. And last, but not least, to Cath for inspiring me to start writing in the first place, coming out with me, keeping me fit and denying me unhealthy food. Apart from the odd chips and ice cream at the seaside. And tirelessly correcting my, incorrect grammer' spelling and: punctuation.

ABOUT THE AUTHOR

Andy Keen

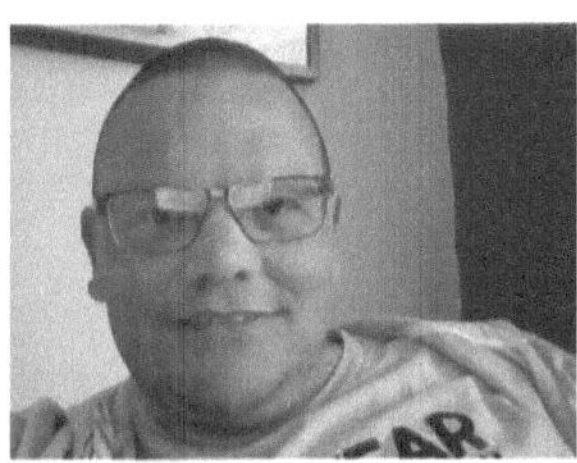 Andy was born in Rugby, the youngest of four children, to a Methodist minister. Their Father died of a heart attack six months later. The family then moved to Cheshire. He was educated at the Methodist Kingswood school in Bath. Andy's brother died when he was 28. Andy had a heart attack and quintuple by-pass in December 2013 whilst living and working in Devon. Andy has three children and now lives and works in Staffordshire. Andy is marrying Cath in Spring 2021. Both Cath and Andy are active members of Rising Brook Community Church in Stafford.

BOOKS BY THIS AUTHOR

Coconuts And Ice Cream

Most people don't travel anywhere via Australia, but Andy did. The Solomon Islands lie in the South Pacific, the villages do not have electricity but have rice and sweet potato in abundance. Everywhere is a canoe ride away. There are creatures that can injury you and cause you pain. Andy battles it all, and still talks in Church meetings each night.
Being part of the party that officially opened the 'Spotlight on Solomons' youth centre, he got to wear flower garlands and 'attacked' by warriors.
Andy even attended Synod, when he wasn't being ill with suspected Malaria. Learned some Pijin. And bought ice cream when he could.
In return the Solomon Islanders showed him just some of the hundred uses they have for the coconut.

Alphabetical Britain

Sometimes life is about the journey and not the destination. In this book, Andy travels the length and breadth of the country, From Alsager to Zulus. Armed only with a train ticket and a timetable. Andy travels from A-Z in alphabetical order. Visiting England, Scotland and Wales; as far South as Redruth, as far North as Inverkip, as far west as Valley, as far East as York.Visiting twenty-four stations in alphabetical order. He finds stations that are open that have no trains, stations that are closed but have several trains, stations that he has to ask the train at especially for him. He rides short one carriage trains, he rides the longest train in Britain, he rides seated trains, he rides sleeper trains. He uses a Harrington Hump, he uses a First-Class Lounge.He stops off at each place, where some provide more to do than others. He has an 'experience' on an industrial estate in Scotland, walks on a viaduct in pouring rain in England and visits the big station in Wales.If you have ever wondered if alphabetical travel can be done, the answer is here. An outstanding example of a pointless journey.

THE END.

www.ingramcontent.com/pod-product-compliance
Lightning Source LLC
Chambersburg PA
CBHW031228250726
48655CB00005B/1857